Modern Aging

Modern Aging

*A Guide for Seasoned Citizens to
Achieve Health, Happiness and Purpose*

Carole Marks

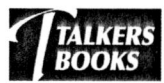

Modern Aging:
A Guide for Seasoned Citizens to Achieve Health, Happiness and Purpose

© 2005 by Carole Marks. All rights reserved.
No part of this book may be reproduced or transmitted in any form or by any means, electronic, mechanical, photocopying, recording or otherwise, or by any information storage and retrieval system, without prior written permission from the publisher, except for brief quotations in critical reviews and articles. For information, please write:
Permissions Department,
Talkers Books,
650 Belmont Avenue,
Springfield, MA 01108 U.S.A.

Books are available for bulk purchase at special discounts.
Special editions or book excerpts can also be created to specifications.
For information, please write: Special Markets Department, Talkers Books.

This publication contains the author's opinions and is designed to provide accurate and authoritative information. It is sold with the understanding that the author, publisher and Focus Communications Inc. are not engaged in rendering legal, accounting, investment-planning, or other professional advice. The reader should seek the services of a qualified professional for such advice; the author, publisher, and Focus Communications Inc. cannot be held responsible for any loss incurred as a result of specific investments or planning decisions made by the reader.

First edition published 2005.
Printed in the United States of America

1 3 5 7 9 10 8 6 4 2

ISBN 1-933118-00-8

Library of Congress Control Number: 2004111835

Published by:
Talkers Books
A Division of Focus Communications, Inc.
650 Belmont Avenue
Springfield, MA 01108

www.talkersbooks.com

Dedication

This book is dedicated to the memory of my parents, Harriet Lehman Marks and Morris F. Marks, Jr. Thank you for all the love and support you gave me over the years, for teaching me the value of honesty, and for believing in my dreams.

And my grandmother, Florence Korn Lehman... the kindest and sweetest human being I have ever known.

I didn't know it at the time, but my catalyst for writing this book was the death in 1996 of both of my parents within three months of each other. I later realized that had they had the right information, the medical traumas that led to their death may have been prevented. Or, at least, they may have suffered far less.

My father was the first to fall ill. On a few occasions his legs buckled under him—classic warning signs of a possible Transient Ischemic stroke—but a doctor assured him he was alright without having initiated a complete work-up for cardiovascular disease. Fast forward several weeks later, when my mother called me to say that my father was feeling tired and was going to stay in bed. She failed to tell me, probably because she was in total denial, that he was so seriously ill and that he was now paralyzed on one side, another indication of a stroke. She therefore didn't think to get him to the hospital and had no idea that there is a golden window of several hours when the proper thromblytic clot-blotting drug could have helped restore blood flow to the brain and possibly prevent some permanent damage. Soon after, my father required round-the-clock care and my mother had to move him to a nursing home.

My mother's precipitous decline started several months later. One day, on her way to visit my father, she fell and broke her hip, requiring hip-replacement surgery. In retrospect, I am sure she had osteoporosis. She was so thin and frail that she lacked both the will and the strength to master walking again. A bit of information—about the benefits of exercise for the elderly, about bone density tests to screen for osteoporosis, and about vitamins and minerals (such as vitamin D and calcium) and medications (such as bisphosphonates and calcitonin)—could have substantially reduced her risk of fractures.

I have sifted through tons of material and interviewed dozens of prominent experts about how to live a long, happy and productive life. Although I wish this book had evolved earlier, so I could have been more informed and helped my own parents live longer and more comfortably, I have made it my mission to help other families make the aging of their parents—and themselves—quite a bit easier. I will have accomplished my mission if this book helps you adopt my mantra... "Getting older means getting better."

Acknowledgements

So many people have helped make this book possible. I offer my deepest gratitude to the following people:

My family brings joy. My grandchildren keep me young at heart. My brother Bob Marks, his wife and family provide an anchor of love and security.

J Scott, my significant other, never fails to deliver ardent support throughout my individual and our joint endeavors.

Shelley Blanchette, my assistant, cheerfully endured all of those 5:00 am meetings.

Michael Harrison, editor and publisher of *TALKERS* magazine, has provided the encouragement and support to see this project through from beginning to end. My other colleagues at *TALKERS* magazine (Kevin Casey, Barbara Kurland, Sharon Harrison and Matthew Harrison) and Talk Radio News Service (especially Ellen Ratner and Victoria Jones) provided a rich infrastructure of information, technical services and cheerleading that were crucial to the incubation of this book. Beverly Santaniello, director of production, *A Touch of Grey*, has devoted her unflagging spirit on and off the air. Jayne Pearl, editor, has brought enthusiasm and skill.

Dr. Robert Butler continues to bring greater public understanding of the aging process and the extension of opportunities for older individuals in our society. His Pulitzer Prize for his book, *Why Survive? Being Old in America*, exemplifies the unusual nature of that talent and contribution.

All the wonderful organizations I worked for including the Retired and Senior Volunteer program have given me the opportunity to serve others and expand my horizons.

The great journalist Helen Thomas has long been a professional role model and inspiration for me.

Amy Hendry, my physical trainer, makes workouts both mentally and physically enjoyable.

Dr. Christopher Morren has stood by me as a physician and a friend and has kept an eye on my health so I may continue to live my life to the fullest.

Introduction

I have witnessed many friends and relatives as they enter their senior years. Some have thrived. For others, it's been truly rough. I've often wondered what differentiates those who gracefully waltz their way through their twilight years from those who fearfully and begrudgingly limp or crawl.

After reviewing my notes from countless interviews of authors and experts in many fields—ranging from celebrities to everyday folks—and researching all the topics that comprise this book, I think I have found the answer.

In Volkswagen commercials the announcer proclaims, "There are drivers and there are passengers." That's true in life, too. Some passengers sit in the back seat and enjoy the view. Some are backseat drivers and are quick to point out the faults in others. Others close their eyes and miss experiencing major portions of the adventure. Some passengers end up in the trunk, bouncing and thrashing with every sharp turn and every bump, along with the spare tire and flying groceries.

Those in the passenger seats never really take charge of where they're going or how they get there. They may not limp or crawl, but neither do they dance much. Sadly, those in the trunk miss all the joy and satisfaction. They feel jostled and jolted through life.

In contrast, those in the driver's seat seem to lead the most meaningful and zestful lives. Because they are steering the car, they take control and responsibility for the direction, duration and side trips of their lives.

My mission in writing this book is to help readers find their way into the driver's seat. How to get started? Here's a little exercise to begin: Imagine you are in the twilight of your years on this planet, looking back at the moments and relationships of your life. What do you hope to see? How will you know if you have led a life that has been meaningful, vital and fulfilling?

Now consider, at your present age and stage of your life, what you need to do more—and less—of, so that when you near the end, you will feel blessed and peaceful.

Perhaps you still have work-related goals you seek to achieve. You're in luck! This book will explore many issues boomers and older workers face in the workplace, including ageism and how to avoid it.

If achieving great health is your major concern, this book offers plenty of ways to take charge of taking care of yourself, plus how to navigate the increasingly complex health-care system.

Some folks may feel fulfilled just to improve the quality or quantity of sex—and guess what? You'll find plenty of frank and thoughtful advice about love, dating and sexual satisfaction.

As well, this book will engage you in a provocative debate about the pros and cons of technology, as it relates to aging boomers and beyond. Devices and tools our parents never heard of can prolong life and make living longer more pleasant, safer, and more rewarding in many areas of our lives. However, some technologies can be difficult for older people to use, and limit some aspects of the way we live, even as they enhance other aspects of our lives.

Whether your hair has just a touch of gray, has gone all gray—or has just plain gone—I've written this book to help us take a long, hard look at some of our most profound needs and wants, and consider ways to meet those needs and wants most effectively.

Growing old has never been so full of choices, opportunities and, of course, challenges. It is my profoundest wish that this book will help seniors and aging boomers grab a set of keys, jump into the driver's seat and put the pedal to the metal, so that when you reflect on these later years, you marvel with pride at how you have confidently navigated your own way through every twist and turn!

"Gray hair is a crown of splendor; it is attained by a righteous life."

- Proverbs 16:31

*"It gives me great pleasure to converse with the aged.
They have been over the road that all of us must travel
and know where it is rough and difficult
and where it is easy and level."*

- Plato

*"Is not wisdom found among the aged?
Does not long life bring understanding?"*

- Job 12:12.

Contents

Chapter 1.	*Truths and Myths of Aging*	1
Chapter 2.	*The Methods to My Media Madness*	9
Chapter 3.	*Making Work Work for You*	21
Chapter 4.	*Best and Worst of Technology*	33
Chapter 5.	*It Ain't Over 'Til It's Over: Dating, Love and Sex Later in Life*	43
Chapter 6.	*DO Try This at Home*	55
Chapter 7.	*Grannies Getting Off Their Fannies: Redefining Grandparenting*	75
Chapter 8.	*How to Afford or Avoid Retirement*	91
Chapter 9.	*Traveling in Style*	103
Chapter 10.	*Live to be 100: How to Take Charge and Take Care of Ourselves*	119
Chapter 11.	*Navigating the Health-Care System*	133
Afterthoughts		147
Resources		149
Notes		167

Chapter 1

Truth and Myths of Aging

In 16th Century Britain and the American colonies, seniors were so respected that younger folks tried to look older by wearing powdered wigs and cutting their clothes to imitate the sloping shoulders of the elderly. Our society has come a long way, but not all for the better. Over the past several decades, "seasoned citizens" have been doing everything possible to hide gray hair, sagging bodies and wrinkled faces. Youth is in, old is out.

But not for long! The 76 million baby boomers born between 1946 and 1964 are bound to change all that as they approach 65—the official onset of senior citizenship. They're not about to get left behind by the youth culture, at least not without putting up a big fight.

In 1990, I had the good fortune to launch a local radio program at WSUB in Groton, Connecticut called *Senior Focus* in which I set out to apply many of the principles I was learning in my life to helping older folks and their families in my community. Clearly, there was a need for such a program and it enjoyed tremendous growth and acceptance.

Today, as host of *A Touch of Grey: The Talk Show for Grownups*, a daily one-hour radio program syndicated to more than 50 stations around the country, my mission remains the same as it was during the early days of *Senior Focus*—to help people approaching or in their senior years identify the main challenges that come with aging. With my regular co-hosts—*TALKERS* magazine editor Michael Harrison; prominent attorney/author Steven J.J. Weisman; and WFAN, New York host Richard Neer; —we cover everything from health care issues to families, housing, work, technology and play.

A little bit about my co-hosts:

Michael Harrison, who helped edit this book, is one of the most prominent behind-the-scenes opinion leaders in the talk radio and TV industries. He is the editor and publisher of *TALKERS* magazine, the leading trade publication in these fields and an expert on American public opinion as it is expressed in the media.

Steven J.J. Weisman is a nationally prominent Massachusetts-based attorney heard for years on Boston's leading talk stations. An acknowledged expert on elder law, Mr. Weisman is the author of *A Guide to Elder Planning: Everything You Need to Know to Protect Yourself Legally and Financially* (Prentice Hall) and executive director of the Internet-based legal resources organization, iLawAmerica.com.

Richard Neer is one of America's best radio sports talk show hosts. He is heard on WFAN, New York and spent years on the New York Giants Radio Network. He is also an accomplished broadcasting generalist whose contemporary cultural roots go back to the early days of FM rock radio. Mr. Neer is the author of *FM: The Rise and Fall of Rock Radio* (Villard).

All three gentlemen are baby boomers who bring a wide range of insight and knowledge—not to mention professional broadcasting skills—to our round table discussions.

We have had an opportunity to interview hundreds of fascinating luminaries on the show from a variety of fields including Jimmy Carter, Hillary Clinton, Madelaine Albright, Billy Crystal, Arlo Guthrie, John McEnroe, Jill Clayburgh, Donna Mills, Mary Chapin Carpenter, Billy Joel, Suzanne Somers, Doris Roberts, Melanie Mayron, Maria Muldour, Ann-Margret, Carl Reiner, Marvin Hamlisch, and Janet Leigh—in addition to terrific doctors, professors, government officials and a wide variety of authors. Together we explore the most important themes and situations of our times from an adult perspective.

This book will address these issues and present how people of the "sixties generation," as they hit their sixties, are bound to redefine aging.

I come to this task with an eclectic background—reflecting the way workers in the 21st century will hold a variety of different jobs, perhaps in a variety of different fields. My work history didn't start until I was in my forties. I married at age 18, before I could finish my first semester at college. I became a stay-at-home wife, raising four children. When my marriage began to disintegrate, I quickly came to realize two things: first, if I got divorced, I would need to support myself; and second, if I wanted a job, I needed to get a college education.

I earned an associates degree in criminal justice and then a bachelor's degree in human services. After being away from the academic world for so many years, I realized that getting older was getting better. I was so eager to learn and so focused that I graduated with a 4.0 average.

At the school that I attended, 95% of the students were African-American or Americans from the island of Puerto Rico. Many of the professors espoused a revolutionary philosophy; a number of them had been actively involved in the Black Panthers movement. While I did not always agree with their militancy, I did find their ideas challenging. They helped me better appreciate and understand other cultures—both their problems and values.

My first jobs out of college involved working with convicted criminals. First, at a pre-trial release program, my job was to get each client treatment, if needed, and a job to help pay their fines. My ultimate responsibility was to see that my clients showed up for their court appearances. My 99% record of finding them and making sure they appeared in court required creativity—and courage!

At my next job, at a halfway house on the grounds of a jail, I found out that most of my clients were quite happy being criminals and were quite smug about their inside knowledge of the criminal justice system. In many cases, they were able to subvert the system and make it work for them. The clients that I actually got into treatment programs and who went on to have a more productive life were few and far between. These were clients who made changes because they wanted to, not because it was mandated by the courts. I have never forgotten this lesson about effecting change.

Eventually, I landed a position as director of a federal program that worked with senior volunteers. Ah, I thought, the only crime this group is guilty of is the one imposed by our youth-worshiping society: getting old. Between 1984 and 1990, I oversaw 750 volunteers who worked at nearly 100 non-profit agencies in 11 towns. Many of my volunteers were very active, lived independently, and were in their 80s and 90s. I began to realize that I was seeing the beginning of a whole new group of pioneers. These active seniors, or seasoned citizens as I like to call them, were operating in uncharted territory: As a demographic group, on average they were living longer than any previous generation. To make the most of their expanded lifetime, I felt they needed all kinds of useful information. For example, in today's world of Medicare, HMOs and rushed medical visits, patients have to be their own health advocates. Every week an enormous number of new medicines, treatments and devices emerge. It's bewildering, and I saw clearly a need for someone to sort through all the news we're bombarded with and tell older Americans what they needed to know to live longer, happier and fuller lives.

Here are some of the most important topics we will cover and myths we will demystify in *Modern Aging*:

Myth: Old age is a direct cause of declining health. Actually, our state of mind and how we take care of ourselves largely determine our physical health. While a positive attitude certainly doesn't guarantee good health, our approach to whatever life hands us profoundly impacts our ultimate destiny.

Myth: Older Americans tend to be pretty much alike. In his book, *The Nine Myths of Aging* (Thorndike Press, 1998), Douglas K. Powell describes the rapid increase in ethnic and racial diversity among the older population. Of course, the spread in physical and mental abilities is fairly wide, too. While some older Americans are declining in health, a significant number can function physically and mentally as well as their younger counterparts.

Myth: Old age and poverty go hand in hand. A little more than 10 percent of this country's elders live in poverty—that's still way too high, but certainly not the majority. The National Council on the Aging says that senior households control half the nation's discretionary income and own three-quarters of all financial assets. They will leave their children and grandchildren an astonishing inheritance of ten trillion dollars in cash and assets.

Myth: The older you get, the more set you become in your ways. In truth, people's vocabulary, conceptual and creative skills often grow after age 60. The fastest growing segment of our population to take up the computer—with relish, I might add—is seniors. Consider that Pablo Casals was giving concerts at 88, Michelangelo was carving masterpieces at 89, and Winston Churchill wrote his book, *The History of the English-Speaking Peoples* (Greenwich House, 1987), when he was 83.

Myth: When you get older, the first thing to go is memory. While some mental capacities, such as spatial skills, processing speed and multi-tasking, do tend to decline, there are many ways to compensate for these skills, which tend to decline before memory.

Myth: Sex drive declines dramatically with age. "Learning and sex until rigor mortis," demanded Maggie Kuhn, the late co-founder of the Gray Panthers. I think she would agree that the traditional pattern of human development (education, work, then leisure/retirement) will be replaced by a new model consisting of education, work and leisure being interspersed repeatedly throughout one's life. It will become normal for 50 year olds to go back to school and for 70 year olds to start new careers.

Now, a couple of truths about aging:

Truth: Today's seniors and soon-to-be boomer geezers have enormous influence in terms of sheer numbers, money and power. Consider:

- People over age 50 currently account for 25% of the U.S. population.

- With 48 million baby boomers turning 50 in 2005, older Americans will be able to determine who the nation's elected leaders will be. They and their organizations such as the American Association of Retired Persons (AARP) will be able to have enormous influence over policy—making, tilting policies in favor of those 50+.

- They earn a combined annual personal income of $800 billion and control 70% of the total net worth of U.S. households-nearly $7 trillion of wealth.[1]

- More than 95 percent of the top-paid CEOs are over age 50 (74% are age 51-60; 22% are 61+).[2]

Despite enormous challenges our aging population must confront, we have an unprecedented opportunity to take control of many aspects of those issues. For example, concerning ageism, boomers will not likely be as passive as many of today's older generation. We will explore how boomers' legacy of activism and their willingness to question authority will affect general attitudes about aging in the media, the work place and on policies.

Truth: Despite our youth-obsessed culture, our leaders seem to be in denial over the growing differences in priorities between younger and older Americans.

The areas where potential intergenerational clashes will most likely occur involve how our country's financial resources will be allocated and the manner in which its citizens will be taxed. Older Americans believe their health and financial security depend on Social Security and Medicare benefits remaining intact. However, while changes to those programs were much needed, the deeply flawed 2003 Medicare Reform Act does nothing to contain future costs of drugs and will curtail some benefits of many low- and middle-income people. In Chapter 11 we'll analyze the effects of the Medicare Reform Act.

Younger Americans, on the other hand, want to be more independent, don't trust the government, and don't want to be strapped with paying taxes for so many retired workers. A well-paying job with good benefits is a top priority. Today's younger workers see that retirees during the past 30 years have done very well economically. They don't believe they will do as well. Another difference comes in the area of education. For young parents, the quality of their children's education is very important. Seniors, on the other hand, sometimes vote down school budgets. Throw in the mix of an uncertain economy, an unbalanced federal budget, and a bloodied stock market, and you might just have the recipe for "intergenerational warfare."

To avoid a future confrontation between working-age taxpayers and the exploding number of retirees they will be asked to support, we must first acknowledge that the young and the old may have different needs at different stages in their lives. The next step is to realize that providing for the largest generation of seniors in history, while simultaneously investing in education and job opportunities for tomorrow's workers, will require major policy changes.

Richard D. Thau, co-author of *Generations Apart* (Prometheus Books, 1997), says that boomer-age politicians will have to make radical fiscal reforms, such as some kind of means testing for the entitlement programs—Social Security and Medicare. When you think about it, we already have means testing in many parts of our life. For example college scholarships, getting a mortgage, property tax relief, and our individual taxes are all based on our individual strengths and weaknesses. Not everyone receives equal treatment. I strongly believe that the fiscal reform for Medicare and Social Security benefits should be called affluence testing. Middle-class and upper-income seniors will have to forgo part of their federal benefits, while benefits to low-income seniors may even be raised. Working Americans will be forced, out of necessity, to save a higher percentage of their income if they want to have a financially secure old age. Americans, who are the world's worst savers, will have to have strong incentives to do this, possibly in the form of tax credits.

In our chapter on health care, we will see how patients can advocate for themselves when doctors prescribe medication, when we are admitted to the hospital or undergoing tests, to make sure our needs and concerns are understood and met. We will learn how we have made important strides in our health consciousness, by smoking less and exercising more. Perhaps our generation will suffer less from lung cancer and joint problems. But challenges remain—we are also eating more, which may account for a dramatic increase in obesity and diabetes.

In our chapter on retirement, we will consider the consequences of a larger portion of boomers who are white collar/professional and are more acquisitive than previous generations (buying every new electronic gizmo, etc., trading in cars every few years and owning second homes and time shares—in other words, spending A LOT), while today's 65+ may have less education and have, on average, a higher proportion of blue-collar jobs and lower income, but spend a lot less, save a lot more, and carry much less debt. We'll focus on the question: How will all this wash out in the coming years?

Indeed, keeping one's body, mind and spirit active goes a long way to helping us feel youthful, even as we age. This book will unearth some of the techniques with which experts and some of our biggest cultural icons are coping with the challenges of getting older, and put those techniques into the context of how the rest of us are managing with our own battles with time, money and nature.

It is my hope that this book will help you fight the many myths of aging, as well as ageism itself. I believe as passionately as ever that, armed with the proper knowledge, getting older can still mean getting better. Read on, to find out how you can avoid driving into the age trap!

Chapter 2

The Methods to My Media Madness

Before I started *Senior Focus* in 1990 at Groton, Connecticut's WSUB radio station, I had been a guest on one of that station's talk shows. At the time, I was director of the Retired Senior Volunteer Program (RSVP) in Groton, and I was invited on the air to discuss what my organization was doing. The interview went so well, I was invited to come in every month and talk about some of the nonprofit organizations where the RSVP's senior volunteers devoted their time.

New Show for Older People

It didn't take long for me to come up with the idea to have a program devoted to the concerns of older people—to provide lots of different information, not just interview nonprofit organizations. So I went to the station manager with the idea. I told him that although it was customary for some people to pay to be on the air, I did not want to do that. Instead, I offered to go out and sell enough advertising to make the show a moneymaker. He took a chance and agreed to give me a one-hour slot from 9:00 to 10:00 in the morning. I got 50 percent of the money from the commercials and the station got the other 50 percent. I did almost everything myself—I went out and sold advertising, booked the guests, wrote the commercials and sometimes recorded them. Just about the only things I didn't do myself were production and engineering. The station provided me with a producer/studio engineer to run the commercials and provide technical help.

When I went out to hit the streets to get advertisers, I found many people who were excited about advertising on a show to reach the upper-demographic market. One of my sales techniques was to invite advertisers or experts at their organizations to come on my show. If it was a hospital, I got doctors to do different segments during the year on medical topics. If it was a drug store, I had a pharmacist who had a good personality talk about side effects or interactions between multiple medications. I was very particular about the advertisers I had on the show, but found plenty.

Targeting Nontraditional Radio Advertisers

My value to WSUB was that I brought in advertisers who had never and would never normally advertise on radio—so-called "nontraditional revenue—from funeral homes, pharmacies, hospitals, and nursing homes. By combining the selling of commercials with the exposing of important people in the community, many local professionals and business people became popular personalities. It was a win-win-win for the station, the advertisers, and me.

My approach helped me identify a giant vacuum, an untapped niche, that includes not only a large segment of the public, which wasn't being served, but a whole advertising community and economy that radio wasn't reaching. As a matter of fact, one day I sat down, put my commercials in order and I figured out I covered everything from getting sick, going to the hospital, getting your medicines, the retirement home, an ambulance company, to your final resting place that all advertised on my show.

As a result, *Senior Focus* became a big money maker. The station manager told me my show had as much advertising as Rush Limbaugh, whose show aired on the station right after mine. It boggled my mind that this all started at WSUB in Groton by me, a mostly self-educated, former housewife! These were heady, exciting times, but a bigger picture and bigger possibilities were beginning to come into focus for me.

After all, while most media in this country are geared to young people and commercial interests, my program, geared to the upper-demographic slice of America, could do as well advertising-wise as the most commercially successful talk show—Rush Limbaugh. My one-hour weekly show evolved into a two-hour show, and then went daily. Eventually, in the mid-1990s, I took the concept of *Senior Focus* national, just as a new development occurred in the radio industry: the explosion of independent syndication. A network called the Talk America Radio Network began to syndicate my show to other stations around the country.

The Joys of Syndication

Talk America Radio Network happened, at that time, to specialize in small, independent, nontraditional-revenue (NTR) shows—and like me, it was geared to selling to people who normally wouldn't advertise on radio. This approach has become a big movement today. The traditional approach is to go to advertising agencies that represent regular advertisers and try to get our share of the pie by selling cost-per-thousand listenership. This is *quantitative* selling. They're selling purely by numbers—attempting to target "x" number of people listening and not caring what they're like—smart or dumb, rich or poor, old or young—just as long as they hear my Coke or Buick commercial.

I was taking a *qualitative* approach, which targets special kinds of listeners who are apt to buy a certain product. I can understand the general mindset of advertisers and media people who want to go where the numbers are. They don't seem to understand that qualitative broadcasting can make more money because its audience is active. Qualitative selling means segmenting your audience, and targeting people who meet certain criteria—perhaps because they like to eat in fine restaurants or enjoy travel, or are interested in the education of their children—that make them more likely to respond to your message.

The beauty of my show is that by gearing programming to older Americans, I had the benefit of it not only being quantitative (some 25% of all Americans are age 50 or older), but also qualitative.

My Fledgling Media Empire Takes Root

Shortly after I began syndicating *Senior Focus* daily on Talk America Radio Network, I launched a little organization, Senior Focus Incorporated, and hired Shelley Blanchette as my right-hand woman and affiliate relations person. She's still with me today.

I based the national show on the model of my show at WSUB, and found there were a number of stations around the country happy to have my program. I began to sell advertising time on a national level the same way I sold to local advertisers, but by now I was going after multinational pharmaceutical companies instead of local drug stores and national insurance companies instead of local nursing homes and funeral homes.

But my major turning point came when I met Michael Harrison, editor and publisher of *TALKERS* magazine, at a national radio industry conference in Los Angeles. I took an instant liking to him. Harrison and the magazine encouraged newcomers to the business and provided the promising ones with exposure. It was unusual because most people aren't open and don't give new people a hand up. I also recognized that his magazine played a major role in promoting the entire talk radio phenomenon. Many people, in fact, believe *TALKERS* was one of the three or four defining elements in the history and evolution of the modern talk radio movement. Harrison galvanized fragmented and isolated talk show hosts by creating a sense of community, by helping them identify their common interests and challenges, and by encouraging people and promoting talk radio to the outside world.

Acquiring *TALKERS* magazine

Harrison and *TALKERS* magazine were so sympathetic to the mission of *Senior Focus* that it led to our becoming partners. I acquired a major ownership stake in *TALKERS* magazine and appointed Harrison president of Senior Focus Incorporated, while I remained chairman. With the addition of *TALKERS* to my company's holdings, we changed the name of the firm to Focus Communications because it was no longer just focusing on seniors—*TALKERS* magazine is about the entire talk radio industry (in addition all of the emerging talk media platforms).

Changes were in store for my show, too. Initially, it was geared to the 60 and 70+ crowd. Harrison broadened the content and the market to include post-war baby boomers, a 76 million-person market that is active, largely upscale and confronting a myriad of issues. With that shift in focus, we renamed the show *A Touch of Grey* (after a Grateful Dead song). Before, my approach had been to address my audience by saying something like, "When you're going to a nursing home, here's what you should watch out for." Harrison shifted that to, "If your parents are going to a nursing home, here's what you should look for." It became more about the active older person than the older person who needs to be taken care of.

I have devoted my resources to *TALKERS* because I believe the magazine, unlike most trade magazines, fosters quality and diversity in media, not just the commercialization of it. *TALKERS* magazine was an enormous success story well before I came along, and I am devoted to helping Harrison broaden its base, just as Harrison is helping me broaden mine. Our partnership, more than anything else, is a manifestation of a warm friendship between us. We share the same values. While it's not *TALKERS*' mission to promote upper-demographic programming (which is the mission of my show), the magazine encourages the industry to have diverse programming. Hence, at *TALKERS* magazine's annual "New Media Seminar" conferences (the industry's major convention) we have urban broadcasting, women broadcasters and specialty broadcasting in addition to mainstream political talk radio.

Through Harrison, I met Ellen Ratner, *TALKERS*' Washington, D.C. bureau chief and founder and president of Talk Radio News Service (TRNS). Ratner, who is known by most of Washington's power elite on a first-name basis, launched TRNS in 1993 as a news agency that, as its name implies, caters primarily to talk radio. I have been watching Ratner ever since she was another struggling female radio talk show host. She was not deterred when she concluded that the industry did not welcome a liberal woman. Instead, like me, she identified and successfully filled a vacuum that the standard news broadcasts to talk radio stations failed to address—the kinds of issues compatible with and targeted to the talk radio audience. For the past decade, TRNS has been presenting the news in the currency of talk radio—conversation itself.

According to Ratner, her fledgling bureau's mission was to provide news to talk radio stations in an interactive style and impact directly on the front porch, back fence and pocketbook issues that are the meat and potatoes of talk radio. TRNS presents news to its affiliates in two ways: straight news without "spin," and news that is laced with opinion. Both entail the "reporter" interacting—even debating—with the local host (plus listener calls), to give the impression that TRNS is that particular station's or network's arm in Washington. Customization is the key.

She began with a staff of one—herself—plus a team of as many as 15 student interns, and proceeded with the difficult process of obtaining Capitol Hill credentials, almost impossible in those days for an organization with "talk radio" in its name. With her team, she could simultaneously cover several Congressional hearings, a Pentagon briefing and a White House news conference as well as demonstrations around town.

In those days, talk radio was not respected by the traditional mainstream news-gathering organizations. And although talk radio still faces some discrimination in the Washington news culture, all talk broadcasters owe Ratner a debt of gratitude for paving the way toward journalistic respect in the nation's capital.

The success of Ratner's strategy is evidenced by the enormous and diverse client base TRNS has attracted over the past decade: the entire political spectrum is represented from the left-wing Free Speech Radio News to the right-wing Radio America. Clients over the years include Fox News Channel (for which Ratner serves as a political analyst), American Urban Radio Network, Radio Wall Street, Talk America Radio Network, and even *TALKERS* magazine, as well as more than 500 individual radio stations around the U.S. and abroad.

Acquisition Number Two: TRNS

I'd been so impressed with Ratner's long list of accomplishments and the sheer force of her intelligence, compassion and fearlessness, that just prior to writing this book, I acquired TRNS and added it to the divisions of Focus Communications. I'm delighted that Ratner will continue to oversee the day-to-day operation of her company in the newly created role of bureau chief. She will also continue as *TALKERS*' Washington bureau chief. Beyond being an amazing on-air radio and television talent, she is one of the hardest-working and most enlightened management figures I have ever encountered. She fits right in with the culture of this feisty, bold firm.

Together, Ratner, Harrison and I have the opportunity to see TRNS take on projects and rise to levels that seemed impossible just a few short years ago.

At the same time, this acquisition ushers me into another adventure—the opportunity to be a credentialed Washington correspondent. I won't make this my full-time work, but I do intend to visit Washington regularly to promote the issues concerning aging boomers and seniors. I've been to numerous White House briefings at which many of the concerns of the 50+ generation are neither brought up nor discussed. I want to take a chance and push the envelope a bit. My mission in D.C. is really the same as it's been on the air—to make people realize that it's in their interest and the country's interest to address these issues (many of which I address in this book). My hope and prayer is that politicians will wake up to the fact that there's media out there geared to older people. Maybe they'll start performing in the interests of older people, knowing someone's watching! TRNS is the vehicle by which I intend to walk into Congress, the Supreme Court and the White House, to ask the tough questions, just like my idol, veteran Washington reporter Helen Thomas, does.

We've been so successful with *TALKERS* magazine, *A Touch of Grey*, Talk Radio News Service and my own business interests, that we now have enormous resources that we can use to promote our altruistic agenda. Our company is not dominated by the profit "anything for a buck" motive. Instead, we operate on the notion of "quality for a buck." We are driven by the notion that we can make a lot of money doing what's right.

Therefore, future plans call for *TALKERS* magazine to continue to be a positive influence on all talk media—talk radio, talk cable, talk television and all of that, as well as to champion the First Amendment. TRNS will continue, as part of its larger mission, to be a commercially successful (with a conscience) voice for older folks as well as diversity within the mainstream of American life. On the air at *A Touch of Grey*, and on the ground in our nation's capital, I will continue to focus my energy and resources to fight the forces of ageism.

As much as I love being part of the media, I recognize that the media have been a breeding ground for ageism. And so I have devoted the rest of this chapter to trying to point out some of what we're up against, and what we can do about it.

Platforms for Fighting Ageism

The most fascinating aspect of the term "ageism" is its recent origins. It was coined in 1968 by Dr. Robert Butler, a prominent geriatric physician who was the first director of the National Institute on Aging. The term defines a negative way of looking at and stereotyping elderly individuals. Ageism is an entrenched phenomenon. You can see it in such commonly used phrases as "over the hill" and don't be an "old fuddy-duddy."

When did ageism begin to rear its ugly head? Early in America's history, family elders held a special place of respect and honor. After World War II, a time of great prosperity resulted in an explosion of births. Our country started to focus its renewed hopes and direct its resources toward the large segment of our population born between 1946 and 1964—the baby boomers. At the same time, as increasingly mobile families moved away from their birthplaces, the value of elders' advice and decision-making power began to fade into the background.

Another reason that ageism has found fertile soil in our youth-obsessed culture is that young people, by not acknowledging the importance and relevance of their elders, can block out their own fears about aging.

With 50-and-older Americans representing the fastest growing segment of our population, the media should have a wide variety of stories to report about this group. Sadly, older Americans are largely ignored by the media, and the little coverage they do get is narrowly focused.

The main topics include Social Security, Medicare, elder abuse, and issues that involve sick and dependent seniors. These topics are, of course, important. But what about covering the 95% of today's active seasoned citizens who are living longer, healthier, and more productive lives than any previous generation? They are redefining everything in our culture from new ways of working in retirement to extending the parameters of middle age. A recent survey by The National Council on the Aging (www.ncoa.org) found that middle age was now defined as between 64 and 72 years old!

One of the main reasons these positive stories rarely emerge has to do with advertising, the lifeblood of both printed and visual medial. Buyers at ad agencies determine what airs on TV and radio, and what publications publish. Those selling advertising tend to be in their twenties and thirties. They don't think they are ever going to get old. Their vision of marketing is promoting anything that is cool. The images of older people and their interests are definitely not considered cool.

In addition, ad agencies and their personnel operate under a lot of false assumptions about the 50+ population, such as that older people are poor and cannot afford to purchase new products or services, even if they want to. The truth, however, is quite different. Ken Dychtwald, Ph.D., author of

Age Wave: How the Most Important Trend of Our Time Will Change Our Future (Bantam, 1990), points out that older Americans control over 70% of the total net worth of U.S. households—nearly $7 trillion dollars of wealth.

Another commonly perpetuated misconception is that seniors are brand loyal and are not interested in trying new products. In fact, people over 70 are the fastest growing segment of computer buyers. They also spend more time shopping on the Internet than the average Internet user does.

These myths affect what we see, hear, and read in our news sources. Newscasts have traditionally attracted an older audience. Advertisers, however, want to target young adults, ages 18 to 34. As a result, you may have noticed that the content of local and national newscasts has been lightened over the last several years, to attract that younger audience.

Even the age of those who report the news has stirred controversy. As Paul Kleyman writes in his Congressional Testimony (September 4, 2002), "Image of Aging in Media and Marketing," newspapers try to dispose of upper middle-aged journalists, irrespective of their expertise, to recruit younger people.

Talk radio traditionally has had a large number of older listeners. They grew up with radio and are comfortable with it. They listen, on average, three and a half hours a day. Yet radio stations, agreeing with their ad agencies, are concentrating on programming they hope will attract the coveted 18- to 34-year old age group.

Finally, in the most watched venue of all—television—unfortunately, the last thing most networks want to be identified with is a large older audience. This has swayed them to cancel very successful shows that had an older audience, such as *Murder, She Wrote* and *Diagnosis Murder*.

There is also a shortage of good roles for older actors. They usually portray a family member who provides comedic relief by perpetuating some of the stereotypes of aging.

Despite so-called "reality TV," I'm amazed at how little of what we see resembles the real world. In TV land, there are very few adults over 50 and a much higher percentage of people under 30 than you'll find in our general population.

There is also gender discrimination in the movies and TV. There are many more roles for older men than there are for older women. When older women are portrayed on TV, their roles present a completely false picture of what an older woman should look like. They do this by using flattering lighting, a variety of lens filters that soften wrinkles, and camera angles that hide extra weight. The average older woman, watching unattainable images of older actresses dance across a screen, can only feel a deep sense of frustration with her own appearance. These false images benefit the beauty companies that sell all those anti-aging products.

These forms of ageism, both overt and subtle, projected by the media have had some severe effects on older Americans. Recently, a 20-year study published in the *Journal of Personality and Social Psychology* reported that older people with positive perceptions of aging lived seven and a half years longer than those exposed to negative images of aging. While the study said the media and its current marketing practices were not solely to blame for promoting ageism, it seems obvious that they contributed substantially to the problem.

What We All Can Do

Older viewers need to write to advertisers and demand that they respond positively to the ongoing longevity revolution, which is going to have a tremendous economic impact on them. The movies and network response to the graying of America should involve producing shows that older Americans want to watch. This also means having more meaningful roles for older actors.

A step in the right direction has been the formation of a group in Hollywood called The Industry Coalition for Age Equity to the Media. One of the group's main goals is persuading the entertainment industry that casting older actors is a key to tapping into the buying power of older Americans.

More reporters need to cover the unique concerns of the sandwich generation, baby boomers and their elderly parents. One of the biggest stories of the 21st century will be the explosive growth of the older American population. As a result, our cultural perceptions of aging will be changed forever.

Other Resources

Articles:

Kelly, Pam, "Ageism's Stereotypes Getting Old," *The Charlotte Observer*, Dec. 12, 2002.

Kleyman, Paul, "Images of Aging in Media and Marketing," Congressional Testimony, Sept. 4, 2002.

Ramirez, Eddy, "Ageism in the Media Is Seen as Harmful to Health of the Elderly," *Los Angeles Times*, Sept. 5, 2002.

Books:

Dychtwald, Ken, Ph.D., *Age Power: How the 21st Century Will Be Ruled by the New Old* (Jeremy P. Tarcher, 2000).

Chapter 3

Making Work Work for You

If you support older people's right to work as long as they continue to be productive, you can consider me your best friend. But if you believe the most experienced workers in any field should be put out to pasture, I might be your worst enemy!

After all, I didn't even enter the work force until I hit my forties and I have no intentions of retiring anytime soon. I know I have as much energy and passion about my work as anyone of any age—and a whole lot more experience than my younger counterparts. In addition to feeling I have a lot to contribute as a professional, I know how much pleasure and meaning I derive from my work.

Besides being illegal (which I will discuss further below), ageism in the workplace is downright stupid and shortsighted. During the recession in the early nineties, many companies' favorite cost-cutting device was nudging out older workers with early-retirement programs. Then, during the recovery, when the economy, job market and stock markets began to heat back up in a frenzy, those same companies realized what a horrible mistake they had made. Not only had they lost many of their most productive and experienced employees, but it was extremely tough to find qualified new hires—and expensive! The cost of recruiting and training new people is extremely high. Also, there are fewer younger workers to choose from.

The pool of workers between 35 and 44 is shrinking. By 2010, their numbers will diminish by more than 10%[1]. At the same time, the pool of older workers, age 55 and older, is on the rise, and will grow 32% by 2010. The upshot: employers who need qualified and experienced people will eventually have to tap older workers.

Yet ageism in the workplace—as well as other areas, such as hospitals, clinics and other health-care providers—is pervasive.

Blasting the Myths

The elderly populations suffer from negative stereotyping more than any other identifiable social group, charges P. W. Dail. She argues that preconceived notions about cognition, physical ability, health, sociability, personality, and work capability perpetuate negative stereotypes about elderly people. Indeed, American culture seems to equate increasing age with decreasing value as a human being.[2]

How did the American culture develop such disregard and disrespect for the elderly? Gerontologists Butler, Lewis and Sunderland[3] suggest the following causes:

- A history of mass immigration, still ongoing, mostly consisting of the young leaving the elderly behind in Europe and Asia.

- A nation founded on principles of individualism, independence and autonomy.

- The development of technologies that demand rapid change and specialized skills.

- A general devaluation of tradition.

- Medical advances that have relegated most deaths to later life, producing a tendency to associate death with old age.

All these have made it difficult to embrace old age itself as a valued and contributory phase of life. But employers aren't the only ones who accept myths, such as that older workers lack energy, are techno-phobic and resist change. In fact, Shelbi Walker, president of Long Beach, California-based Back to Work, Inc., a career management agency for 50-plus job seekers, says that older workers buy into these stereotypes, too, and when they approach potential employers, their feeling useless and depleted comes through. Walker is on a mission to convince them, and employers, about the value of older workers. "No other generation that's living today has gone through the transitions, changes and adjustments in this world as older workers," she insists. She puts job seekers and corporate clients looking to hire quality employees through a "timeline exercise" to help them appreciate the value of older workers.

In this exercise, Walker divides participants into small groups and assigns each group a 20-year period from 1900 through 2000. Each group lists all the political, personal, technological, economic, social and cultural changes they can recall experiencing in that period. Then the groups come together and read the list they've created. "This exercise helps them begin to realize and appreciate the changes they have had to live through and adapt to," says Walker. "They remember when computers that used to be size of a room are now size of your palm. They are the only generation that's had to go through these changes. Especially the way the world is today, with so much uncertainty, it's imperative that companies tap into their knowledge base and appreciate their ability to adapt to so much change."

An AARP Career and Work study[4] found that 69% of older workers plan to work in some capacity during their retirement years. Many have to work. Some must support aging parents or adult children who have had trouble "making it" on their own. And as we mention in the chapter on grandparenting, a growing number of seniors are now caring for and supporting their grandchildren. The top seven reasons that respondents to the AARP study say they will continue to work include:

- Need the money, 76%

- Enjoy working, 76%

- Save for retirement, 67%

- To feel useful, 66%

- Maintain health insurance, 65%

- Qualify for Social Security, 48%

- Support family members, 46%

As you can see, five of these seven reasons are related to financial need. Many have had to postpone retirement after the stock market bubble popped in 2001, wiping out much of their retirement savings. "That will keep some working to rebuild their savings and to give the market time to recoup," according to the Dec. 27, 2002 *Kiplinger Letter*. "In addition, the retirement age to get normal benefits under Social Security is gradually being raised. Those born in 1960 or later must retire at 67 to get normal benefits."

Traditionally, the unemployment rates of older workers has been three to six points lower than the overall unemployment rate. "Older workers are much less likely to quit or be thrown out of a job because most companies use a tenure system when they have to do layoffs—the last hired, first fired," says Susan Houseman, senior economist of the Upjohn Institute for Employment Research in Kalamazoo, Michigan. Between 1983 and 1992, the average gap between job seekers 65 and older and the general population was 3.8 percentage points. But that gap has been shrinking dramatically. Between 1993 and 2002, it was only 1.8 percentage points. Houseman suggests that when workers who have retired jump back into the workforce, they've lost their tenure, and are having a tough time finding another job. The tight job market in the post-tech bust has undoubtedly made it especially hard for older people to find or advance in jobs.

An AARP study found that 67% of older workers believe that age discrimination continues to limit their chances for advancement and well being in the workplace. A recent HotJobs.com poll found that 87% of respondents thought an interviewer had held their age against them during a job interview. "Age discrimination continues to damage our society, reducing both the incomes and the self-confidence of millions of Americans," concludes the Administration on Aging report, "Age Discrimination: A Pervasive and Damaging Influence." [5] The report points out, "Age discrimination is sometimes allowed to continue with surprisingly little protest because of long-held assumptions that it is right and proper for older workers to move aside to make room for younger workers who need to support families, that older workers are less competent, and that there's no mileage in training them for new jobs."

The report continues, "In fact, for a variety of reasons, older workers have been leaving the labor force. The percentage of men 55 to 64 in the work force declined from 87% in 1950 to 67% in 1996, and for men 65 and older, from 46% to 16%. The percentage of women 55 and older in the work force hasn't changed substantially because the dramatic rise in the number of women working has offset the increase in early retirements."

A 1992 Louis Harris survey found that 5.4 million older Americans—one in seven of those 55 and older who were not working at that time—were willing to work but could not find a suitable job. Yet, another 1992 Harris survey of 400 companies found that only one in eight companies sees an urgent need to respond to the aging of the work force. Just one in three offers older workers the chance to transfer to jobs with less responsibility and only one in five offers phased retirement.

I find it surprising that there is so much age discrimination in the workplace, considering that the vast majority of CEOs are 50 and older. Almost 80% of CEOs on the Forbes 500 list of public companies are 50 and older, while more than 27% are 60 and older. Even though many of them may feel pressure to step aside, they still wield lots of power in their organizations and certainly many could do more to make sure that at the very least their companies do not discriminate against older workers. I'd think they might even have a vested interest in seeing that their companies create senior-friendly recruitment, advancement, compensation and benefit policies and practices. To the extent that older workers' perceptions of age discrimination are accurate, employers in those places of work are simply breaking the law.

The Law

The Age Discrimination in Employment Act (ADEA), passed in 1967, prohibits work-related age discrimination for Americans 40 and older. The law has some drawbacks, though. For instance, the ADEA does protect job applicants from refusal of employment solely on the basis of age, but it does not apply to elected officials or independent contractors.

In 2002, the Equal Employment Opportunity Commission (EEOC) received 19,921 filings charging alleged age discrimination, a 14.5% increase from the year before.

One such case was leveled against Monsanto Company, based in St. Louis, Missouri, in 1993, after executives in their twenties fired 66 sales managers, 59 of whom were 40 or older. Forty-three of them sued Monsanto. In June 1996, they won, and each plaintiff received $125,000 to $500,000.

Another case concerns more than 150 television writers, who filed 23 state lawsuits in 2002 against television networks, studios, production companies and talent agencies. The plaintiffs based their case on statistical evidence that they have been systematically "gray-listed." For instance, writers older than 50 comprise nearly one-third of the membership of the Writers Guild, a union representing 11,000 writers in the U.S., yet writers 50 and older only accounted for 13 percent of TV writing staffs. Two out of three prime-time series did not have even one writer older than 50 on staff.

The ADEA law, though, also has little "bite"—enforcement is often anemic because overt age bias is so difficult to prove and because the EEOC has such a large backlog of complaints to investigate. Most cases are eventually dismissed for lack of solid evidence of outright bias.

The upshot: in most cases, it's up to us to break any age barriers we encounter.

Countering Ageism, Latent and Blatant

Increasingly, senior job seekers are learning how to turn negative stereotypes on their head with carefully written resumes and by thinking through answers to interviewers' questions. These resumes and interview responses show evidence that predict future performance—rather than simply focusing on a laundry list of past work experience. A dynamic resume should communicate a sense of purpose, professionalism, competence and enthusiasm, says Shelbi Walker, of Back to Work, Inc.[6]

It's also crucial to overcome common misconceptions about older workers—for instance, that you're too slow to survive in a fast-paced work environment or that you lack specific experience in a new field. Your resume should make it clear that your skills, experience, work ethic and perspective are assets that set you apart from other candidates.

For instance, Roberta Chinsky Matuson, principal, Human Resource Solutions in Northampton, Massachusetts, points out, "Age discrimination is real. So the more seasoned job seeker needs to figure out how to write a resume that doesn't close the door on them before they have a chance to even get in the game." Here's what she recommends:

- **Take the age spots out of your resume.** Create a functional resume that clusters your skills, versus a chronological resume that emphasizes years of work history and job titles. While you are at it, update your interviewing wardrobe so that you appear to be more in line with the times.

- **Use your age as an advantage.** Older workers have a perceived value of having a strong work ethic and are known for their ability to be team players. Provide employers with specific examples of situations that play on these strengths.

- **In good times and in bad times, success sells.** Organizations are always looking to buy skills and successes with the hopes that candidates will repeat these moves in their organizations. As a job seeker, be prepared to communicate the value you bring to the organization rather than reading what's on your resume. Write down all of your great success stories and be prepared to share these stories with the interviewer. Describe ways you can utilize these same skills to help the hiring company achieve their goals.

- **Grease your networking gears.** "Who you know" still matters when you search for a job. If your network is rusty, this is the time to apply some oil to get it going again. Now, more than ever, you need to get your foot in the door. Make a list of former bosses and co-workers, consultants you worked with or hired, neighbors who work in industries of interest to you, alumni and professional association colleagues to start making contacts. If they are unable to assist you with your job search ask them for leads. Remember, the squeaky wheel gets the grease. When you do land your new job, don't forget to thank your network for their support and assistance during your job search. People always like to hear about happy endings.

It is equally important to know what a prospective employer is looking for. Research the company's products, services, strategy and culture. You can learn a lot from a company's website. Use this information to position your own skills.

During an interview, be prepared for some tough questions[7], such as:

You seem overqualified for this position. Won't you get bored? <u>Your answer</u>: I can hit the ground running and you'll save money on less training time.

Can you keep up with a company on the fast track? <u>Your answer</u>: I've stayed on top of developments in the industry and I'm computer literate. Plus, I have more energy than ever, now that my children are grown and living away from home!

There is good news for older Americans looking for work, even during economic slowdowns. The Internet makes searching for a job much easier—there are "job boards" where job seekers can post their resumes and online classified ads where employers list their openings. You can search for jobs by industry, job function, company size or geographic region. Online job boards are most helpful for lower-level jobs, but you can also use the web to find out about job openings at all levels at local companies, as an increasing number of organizations list on their websites positions they are trying to fill.

Older job seekers have one major advantage over their younger counterparts: bigger networks of people in your industry and profession. As much as half to 75% of successful job searches depend on networking—calling colleagues and contacts you worked with in and out of the companies where you've worked over the years (including co-workers, managers, people you've supervised, suppliers, and customers), according to Jim Boros, owner of Chicago-based outplacement firm Spherion. Boros says that the higher the salary level, the more important networking is to a successful job hunt.

Boros says that while it can take seven or eight months for a medium- to high-level job seeker to land a position, one woman he recently helped bounce back from being laid off from her job as director of marketing took just two and a half months. She came to his office every day with lists of people to call and visit. Her energy and willingness to contact everyone she knew throughout her career helped her identify opportunities she may have never otherwise found.

Another positive is that there is much less stigma today to having gaps on your resume. If you want or need to return to work after having tried retirement, or if you were laid off from a job, you don't need to feel uncomfortable about how that will look on your resume. You are in excellent company. Economic ups and downs, corporate acquisitions and reorganizations, and increasing bankruptcy rates, as well as family crises, have made it more common for people in all industries, functions and levels to experience one or more bouts of unemployment.

The trick is to emphasize to potential employers how you have turned those circumstances into learning experiences. Perhaps you took a course to refresh your computer skills, mentored a young person, did volunteer work, or cared for an ailing relative. Point out how this period of your life illustrates your loyalty, discipline, energy and ability to deal with adversity.

One of the single most important aids in finding a job is attitude. The extent to which you are able to project an image that you are confident, cheerful and easy to get along with, can make or break a job search.

Finding Senior-Friendly Companies

At many companies, you won't need to work so hard to break through barriers of ageism. You may want to consider applying for a job at one of AARP's 15 best companies for workers over 50. What makes them such great places for older employees to work? The most frequently cited tool to attract and keep older workers is additional flexibility with full benefits. These companies make older workers feel valued and welcome:

ABN AMRO North America, Inc.

Adecco Employment Services

Baptist Health South Florida

CALIBRE

DaVita Inc.

Howard University

Mitretek Systems, Inc.

New York Life Insurance Co.

Principal Financial Group

Prudential Financial

QUALCOMM, Inc.

The Aerospace Corporation

Hartford Financial Services Group, Inc.

The Stanley Group

Ultratech Stepper

Here are the criteria AARP used to judge the companies it selected:

• **Creative recruiting**, such as education benefits to train people to do jobs in areas where there are shortages of qualified workers.

• **Flexible benefits**, such as fewer hours, working from home or a customized schedule.

• **Age-friendly culture**, such as mentoring programs that match younger and older workers, seminars for managers on age diversity in the workplace and training for employees of all ages.

• **Fair compensation**, based on industry norms.

• **Retirement on your terms**, with retirement benefits that allow employees to retire as early as 55 or stay as long as they want to and can produce, and opportunities to ease into retirement with part-time or per-diem work.

In addition, demographic shifts may make more and more companies offer help with elder care. For instance, some employers can help employees purchase long-term care insurance for their aging parents and themselves. Generous leave-of-absence policies are another great benefit for employees of all ages, who may want to take time off for everything from maternity or paternity to caring for aging parents.

The most important thing to remember when it comes to working or looking for work, is that you bring unique qualifications and experiences to the workplace. Hold your head up high and approach employers and colleagues with confidence and good humor. Never sell yourself short!

Other Resources:

Administration on Aging, U.S. Dept. of Health and Human Services
www.aoa.gov
202-619-0724
AoA Legal Services Hotlines in 12 states:
202-619-1058 or 202-619-3951

American Association of Retired Persons (AARP)
Applied Gerontology Group/ Economic Security and Work Issues Section:
202-434-2277
Legal Advocacy Group/Litigation Unit at AARP:
202-434-2060
"How to Stay Employable: A Guide for Midlife and Older Workers"

Equal Employment Opportunity Commission
For information on age discrimination and the Age Discrimination in Employment Act:
www.eeoc.gov
800-669-EEOC
Charge of Discrimination form:
www.jhllp.com/EEOC%20charge_of_discrimination.htm

National Academy of Elder Law Attorneys
www.naela.com
520-881-4005
NAELA promotes improvement in substantive law, legal education and ethical guidelines in serving older persons and serves as a key public policy advocate on behalf of older persons. Also provides online publication, *Questions and Answers When Looking for an Elder Law Attorney*.

Workplace Fairness
www.workplacefairness.org
A non-profit organization that provides information, education and assistance to individual workers and their advocates nationwide and promotes public policies that advance employee rights.

Chapter 4

The Best and Worst of Technology

Technology is a double-edged sword. On the one hand, medical advances have prolonged and greatly improved the quality of our lives. However, the explosion of innovation in communications, computers, transportation, entertainment and the Internet are often inaccessible to the fastest-growing segment of our population—aging baby boomers and seniors.

"Therein lies the paradox," writes Joseph Coughlin, who teaches policy and management at the Massachusetts Institute of Technology, where he leads Age Lab, an initiative on technology and aging. "After spending billions to achieve longevity, we have not made equitable investments in the physical infrastructure necessary to ensure healthy independent living in later years." [1]

Age Lab's mission is to help researchers, business and government "extend the quality of life and provide services, products and technologies that help people maintain their vitality and remain productive," says Dr. Coughlin.

Personally, I approach technology from a purely pragmatic point of view: I'm not afraid to try new gadgets and gizmos, and I am naturally curious about almost everything. But I'm not turned on by technology for technology's sake. I tend to focus on devices and software that can help me stay informed, organized and productive.

My PC with a broadband Internet connection allows me to read various online publications (*The Wall Street Journal*, *The New York Times*, *Los Angeles Times*, *Washington Post* and *Slate*, among others) and to conduct online research. Sometimes I shop on the Internet, though I still prefer catalogs and calling toll-free numbers so I can ask questions. Of course, I have come to depend on e-mail to communicate with colleagues, friends and family. I couldn't even tell you my cell phone number without looking it up because I rarely use it—I keep it in my car for emergencies.

But as the years go by, I confess I have developed a love-hate relationship with my computer and other electronic gizmos. As indispensable as technology has become to my writing and keeping up with news and information related to my *A Touch of Grey* radio show, it can also be incredibly frustrating—and not just when the computer screen freezes and you lose data you just spent hours working on.

A Blessing or a Curse?

Sue Coppola, clinical associate professor of occupational science at the University of North Carolina (Chapel Hill), agrees. She is not so sure technology is the panacea for healthy, independent living. Prof. Coppola warns that our society's increasing reliance on technology can have quite negative physical and emotional consequences:

- **Use it or lose it.** "We are actually accelerating the aging process when we use the remote control for our TVs, or when we drive everywhere and pull up close to the building. There is a decline in physical activity and the debilitation associated with it is turning out to be a much larger factor in terms of physical decline than we ever realized."

For instance, by prescribing a scooter to allow a nursing home patient to get to the dining room and activity room with a lot of ease will increase the immediate quality of life, but at the risk of increasing his or her longer term rate of decline in physical function.

"I suspect the same thing could happen with regard to cognitive devices—as we learn to use calculators instead of doing calculations, our mind declines. Our mind is a muscle. Use it or lose it," explains Prof. Coppola. Another example: programmable cell phones and personal digital assistants such as Palm Pilots mean we don't have to remember phone numbers. "That's why people who do crossword puzzles tend to maintain a little bit better cognitive information," she adds.

- **Creator or destroyer of isolation?** A lot of technology attempts to fill an empty void in people's lives. It gives them something to do and keeps them learning, and enables them to be remotely connected to their loved ones. But always being hooked up can become addictive.

Having tech-free time is a very important part of mental health. While it is true that the computer can minimize isolation, it is also true to the extent that electronic communication substitutes for human touch, we may actually end up more isolated.

Some older people who need supervision—particularly those with dementia—are monitored by video in their rooms, for safety. But not only does that sacrifice a lot of their privacy, it also may result in less human contact, as nurses and aides feel less need to check on them as frequently.

• **Simplifier or complicator of daily life?** Another problem is that new devices may simplify some aspects of our life, but they have many features some users may find difficult to learn. As devices get smaller and smaller, older people with visual or motor difficulties may find them tough to use—the buttons may be too small to see or manipulate, screens may be too high for wheelchair-bound folks to see.

Most electronic devices simply were not designed with older users in mind. Everything from computers, Internet sites, personal digital assistants (PDAs), television remote controls and cell phones were mostly designed by younger people for younger users. So many cars, kitchen appliances and alarm clocks now depend on digital technology that it's hard to escape the increasing demands on regular consumers to acquire the knowledge, comfort and dexterity to be able to drive to town, set the alarm clock or fry an egg.

Harnessing the Best of Technology

Boomers will also redefine the aging process. Not only are they generally more comfortable with technology than the current 65+ set, but "As boomers get a lot of experience with managing their aging parents, we are wising up about how to plan for aging ourselves," says Prof. Coppola. She points out that with many of their parents living well into their nineties and one-hundreds, boomers are learning and pioneering how to adapt to life and going on despite changes in physical and mental abilities.

Designers, media and the business world seem to be waking up finally to the realization that older people may confront one or more impediments to using computers and other electronic devices. Some companies are catching on, and they're finding that features that make products easier to use for older people also appeal to the younger crowd. For instance, Oxo cutlery grips were designed for use by people with arthritic hands, but the products have become popular among young professionals as well.

"If you build something for adults that is easy to use, read and see, guess what? You're benefiting everyone else too," says the Age Lab's Coughlin. For instance, he points out that automakers are beginning to realize the importance of figuring out how to adapt technology (in areas such as night vision, collision avoidance and navigation) to help older adults drive safely for as long as possible. The Renault Twingo is easy to get in and out of and has large dials. Renault's web site also emphasizes the Twingo is "...synonymous with fun, youthfulness, a sense of adventure and a wise simplicity."

Many innovations certainly help compensate for declining visual and motor abilities, says Prof. Coppola. In many cases, applying technology solutions can make it possible for people to continue living in their homes, keep their jobs, and utilize public transportation and other facilities. The Americans with Disabilities Act (ADA), which has helped make transportation, telecommunications, public facilities and the workplace accessible to people with disabilities, is paving the way for older adults who can qualify under the ADA to demand "reasonable accommodation." These include adaptive devices such as computer screens with larger letters at work to enable them to function in these environments.

"People with disabilities have given older populations a huge gift—the right to participate in life through having environments that are flexible to people's needs," says Prof. Coppola.

Computers and the World Wide Web

The Nielsen Norman group has studied usability of the web for seniors and found that "current web sites are twice as hard to use for seniors as they are for younger users." Many web sites freeze their type faces at a small size and override the browser's ability to enlarge font size. Low-contrast color schemes on many sites exacerbate the problem, as do pull-down menus that require a high degree of dexterity.

Although seniors may not be as easily intimidated by technology as many experts think, they do exhibit some skepticism about their electronic experiences. For instance, AARP research has found significant evidence that they worry about privacy and fraud. In fact, some usability problems and design flaws seem to feed those fears and ultimately result in many missed opportunities for online merchants and businesses. For instance, Forrester Research says that on average, web sites lose about half of their potential sales as the result of an inability of users to find what they came to the site for.[2]

But today's older crowd is far from Luddites when it comes to technology. "The idea that older people are techno-phobic is a myth; the real problem is not having the right learning environment," says Laurel Murphy, chair of the AARP Oregon Computer Action Team. AARP volunteers and chapter members across the country are busy helping the 50-plus population grow more comfortable with technology. In many classes developed by various local AARP chapters, older students learn about e-mail, the Internet and chat rooms. In many communities AARP folks are helping to install computers in nursing homes and serving on state technology task forces. And that's just to name a few activities.

AARP estimates that 40% to 50% of U.S. adults age 50 and older have computer access, mostly for going online to e-mail friends and relatives, make purchases, do banking, trade stocks, read publications and search for information.[3] However, many designers of hardware, software, personal electronics and the Internet harbor misconceptions that hinder older people. For instance, some common myths are that older users have limited budgets, limited interests and limited computer skills, and that they just don't use the web.

Ain't so. The so-called "digital divide," based on age, to the extent that it existed in the early days of the World Wide Web, has certainly fizzled. In 1997, considered the year the web began to proliferate among the general populace, the U.S. Department of Commerce estimated that people 55 and older did have the lowest online access (8.8%) of any segment.[4] However, just two years later, seniors became the fastest-growing demographic group on the Internet, according to Media Metrix, a prominent firm that measures web usage.

More than three-quarters of older adults have taught themselves to use the Internet, and almost half have been online for more than five years, estimates SeniorNet, a nonprofit organization that provides education for and access to computer technology and the Internet to older adults, operating more than 220 learning centers across the United States.

Another study, by Yankelovich Monitor in 2002, found that the most frequent uses of the internet of Americans ages 40 to 64 include:

- 87%   E-mail
- 63%   Just surfing
- 61%   Reading news
- 60%   Getting directions/maps
- 58%   Personal research
- 54%   Travel information
- 46%   Accessing health or medical information
- 33%   Purchasing airline tickets
- 30%   Checking bank account transactions
- 26%   Accessing stock quotes
- 19%   Accessing insurance information
- 13%   Making financial transactions

"We all talk about older people being afraid of technology. I think that's not really true," says Whitney Quesenbery of Whitney Interactive Design, LLC, a consultancy in user-centered design, interface design and usability. The former principal and senior vice president of design at Cognetics Corporation explains, "What happens, as you get older, is you use the technology you're comfortable with and your habits are more deeply formed. But I have colleagues who took up PCs when they turned 70."

One reason more and more seniors are logging online is that companies such as Microsoft are making the Internet cheaper and easier to use, with services such as MSN TV service (877-932-8857; www.msntv.com), which allows users to access the Internet and e-mail through their regular television sets. MSN TV, which costs less than $100, consists of a small receiver that sits atop a TV and connects it with a phone line.

Even people with visual or hearing challenges can access the web. An increasing number of web sites (including my own: www.atouchofgrey.com) are "Bobby-approved." Bobby tests web sites for compliance with government standards, including the U.S. Government's Section 508,[5] and suggests how such sites can meet the Web Content Accessibility Guidelines provided by the World Wide Web Consortium's (W3C) Web Access Initiative.

For instance, for the visually impaired, a Bobby-approved web site would convert its written content into an audio version. I felt strongly that if I was representing my radio show and web site as places where aging Americans can get information to make their lives better, it should be accessible by people with handicaps. I also concur with Tim Berners-Lee, the inventor of the World Wide Web, who has said, "The power of the web is in its universality. Access by everyone regardless of disability is an essential aspect."

Techno Tips

Prof. Coppola offers the following tips that can help us harness the best technology has to offer in the most effective way:

1. Be flexible about how you accomplish tasks. For instance, a person who loves gardening doesn't have to give that up the moment arthritis sets in. But she would be wise to find different ways to pursue this passion without bending on her knees for hours, to avoid exacerbating her condition by further inflaming and overstressing joints and surrounding tissue.

Some ways to work within her new limitations might include researching new-fangled gardening stools, tools with long handles to give her other ways than on her hands and knees. She can also, of course, plant a smaller garden, create a raised garden she can weed and prune without bending, or enjoy house plants more.

If you love reading but your vision has decreased due to macular degeneration, there are lots of devices that can help, such as a computer screen that can enlarge writing, or books on tape. Prof. Coppola suggests thinking about occupations and activities you enjoy and what's important about them and be willing to do them differently.

2. Educate yourself on what resources there are. For instance, check into devices—from low-tech things such as a reaching device if you have back trouble and can't pick up something off the floor or reach a high shelf, to what kind of computer system is right for your home.

Consider inviting a local geriatric occupational therapist to speak at your church or synagogue, senior center, Parkinson's or arthritis support group, about the latest approaches and technologies for enhancing independent living.

3. Be skeptical about devices. There are copycat "knock-offs" of just about every type of device, many of which simply don't work as well as the original. Some people who are relatively able-bodied and sharp of mind may be able to adapt to a lower quality version of an assistive device, but in many cases you really need just the right thing to get the result you want. For instance, there are dozens of different types of reachers. Someone with minor back trouble may do well with a bottom-of-the-line reacher. But another person with poor balance or vision may need a different type of device for reaching high cabinets. Even though reachers seem simple, there are a lot of nuances that make a huge difference as to whether it will be useful.

How do you know which version of any device is right for you?

First, be clear on which problem you're trying to solve. People sometimes get things that seem cool but may not really solve the problem. Base your selection on specific needs.

Second, demand an opportunity to try out a device before you buy it. If you like to shop over the Internet, make sure the online store offers a good return policy.

4. Make sure you shop at reputable stores. For low-cost medical devices, for example, you can order North Coast Medical's catalog at 800-235-7054 (or surf over to www.ncmedical.com and click "Functional Solutions Catalog," to view a picture of a sampling of devices (bath and hygiene products, cushions, dining, eating equipment, mobility devices, canes, etc.) from its catalog. Another good sources is the American Occupational Therapy Association's "Buyer's Guide" (877-404-AOTA).

When it comes to devices that require service, stick with trusted retail stores that offer a service component.

5. Consider the context—where you will be using a device. If you travel, for example, you may want to purchase portable devices when available, such as a folding bath chair you can take to a hotel. Think about all the places you might want to use your devices.

Other Resources:

Access America for Seniors
www.seniors.gov
One of several projects created at the direction of the National Partnership for Reinventing Government (NPRG). Access America is former Vice President Gore's project to get Americans connected to government services via the Internet. The Social Security Administration (SSA) agreed to create, host and maintain AAS as a service especially geared toward senior citizens.

Age Lab, Massachusetts Institute of Technology
www.web.mit.edu/agelab
A partnership with industry and the aging community to develop new technologies promising healthy, independent living throughout the human lifespan. Its research focuses on engineering, computer science, human factors, health and medical sciences, management, marketing and the social and behavioral sciences.

Agilent Technologies
www.americangeriatrics.org
From optical and wireless communications to disease and discovery

research, Agilent delivers product and technology innovations that benefit millions of people around the world.

Design and Usability Testing Center, Bentley College
http://ecampus.bentley.edu/org/dutc/
A not-for-profit enterprise that offers the local software, hardware, and web development communities the independent research and testing resources they need to secure competitive advantage in an increasingly tight marketplace.

Gerontological Society of America Formal Interest Group "Technology and Aging"
www.gsa-tag.org
Focused on investigating and applying the results of rapid advances in technology to better the lives of the growing number of older persons in a world-wide society.

Wired Seniors
www.wiredseniors.com
Gives seniors a "Web of Your Own" and serves as the Main Hub of the many Seniors Related Web Sites that makes up the WiredSeniors.com Network and its wide variety of seniors oriented information and programs.

Chapter 5

It Ain't Over 'Til It's Over:
Dating, Love and Sex in the New Millennium

Let's be perfectly frank. Baby boomers created the youth revolution as well as the sexual revolution. They may no longer be card-carrying youth, but many of us 50 and older are certainly not willing to give up our membership in the sexual revolution. But that doesn't mean dating, love and sex are quite the same as in the "peace, love and tie-dye" days of the 1960s.

In a 2000 study, the National Council on Aging found that among respondents 65 and older, 68% say having a sexual relationship will be important in making their later years "meaningful and vital."[1] In another study, nearly half of all Americans 60 and older have sexual relations at least once a month, and 40% want it more often. But Dr. Saul Rosenthal, author of *Sex Over 40* (Jeremy P. Tarcher, 2000), told the Lakeland, Florida, *Ledger* that he thinks the numbers are considerably higher. "I think people over 60 have sex much more often than once a month," Rosenthal said. "Most seniors I know are having sex once a week probably."[2]

About three-fourths of the NCOA study's respondents of all ages believe that a 75-year-old (man or woman) can be considered sexy. Indeed, a whole lot of seniors are still steaming up their bedroom windows. Gray hair, wrinkles and even flab may not be the stuff of most torrid romance novels and movies, but increasingly, movies and other media are focusing on the sexuality of the senior set.

In the somewhat weird movie, *Never Again*, Jeffrey Tambor's paunchy, pudgy 54-year-old character, Christopher, has exclusively dated 25-year-old glamour girls, but begins to question his sexuality after several months of erectionless encounters. He's instantly cured when he meets 54-year-old Grace, played by Jill Clayburgh.

The more years we've lived, the more baggage we come with—and the more baggage future companions come with as well! We are likely to be more bound up in our ways. Jill Clayburgh, for instance, explains to

Christopher, when she first meets him, that she hasn't had sex in seven years, because "Men are big babies and I don't want to take care of them anymore."

When Jill Clayburgh was a guest on *A Touch of Grey*, she mentioned that movie critics Ebert & Roper got into a heated argument about the core issues of the movie. While Roper loved the movie, Ebert complained that it was too sexual—that gratuitous sex took away from the nature of the story.

"I find that so ridiculous—it's not graphically sexual. You don't see a breast," Clayburgh told my radio show listeners. "I don't want people to think this is sweating, panting sex. It's very humorous and bawdy, but not graphic. It celebrates the sexuality of older Americans.

"People just want older people to be romantic and nice. This movie explores sexual fantasy, things you might think about but not do, things you might do. It doesn't limit what is possible for people in their fifties emotionally or sexually in any way."

I agree. I also thought the movie was realistic in its portrayal of the problems people have coming from not having had a relationship in a long time. How traumatizing it is to have to deal with those things. *Never Again* is often the feeling we have, because we realize being involved with someone else can cause us pain.

Yet in my own experience, the desire for companionship, romance and even sex has not diminished an iota as I've advanced in years. I can't speak for everyone, of course. Some seasoned citizens are content to leave the world of romance and sex. But even if you still feel vital and sexual, you're bound to find new and different challenges as you pursue your passion.

Whether you are married, widowed, divorced or single, this chapter will explore the more intimate issues we face with aging.

The Body's Willing, But the Mind Is Hung Up

"Dr. Ruth" Westheimer, the famous sex therapist, told listeners of my radio show that sex is 99% what you have and only 1% what other people think you have. By "what you have," she wasn't referring to muscles and curves. "Okay, you don't look anymore like 25 or 30, but experience and a twinkle in the eye—that's what it's all about," she said with her famous giggle.

The plus-sized Kathy Bates had quite a twinkle in her eye when, playing a flamboyant, eccentric bohemian in the movie *About Schmidt*, she (seemingly) unselfconsciously shed her robe on screen and lowered her buck-naked bod into a hot tub in a (sadly unsuccessful) attempt to seduce a shocked Jack Nicholson. Hooray that Hollywood has presented an older, but heavier, woman as a sexual being.

I suppose if we haven't learned by our fifties and beyond that attitude, humor, intelligence and kindness can be a turn-on to the opposite sex, we never will. But media messages are mighty hard to escape, glorifying images of youthful perfection. Even if you've been married to or living with the same person for decades, confidence in your sexual appeal can wane. And that can prematurely diminish your libido. Let's face it, it's hard to have an orgasm while sucking in your stomach for fear you'll appear fat. And it's tough to maintain an erection when you worry if you're big enough, or if you can still get hard enough.

The lengths to which people go to hang on to their youthful appearance is big business. Botox, plastic surgery, his-and-her implants (silicon breasts and penile pumps), creams and pills may delay the inevitable for a while—at a steep price. But at some point we are going to have to make peace with our maturing flesh and call on our less physical charms and our creativity to sustain us in the bedroom.

In addition to possible feelings of self-consciousness about our changing bodies, older people may find themselves grappling with guilt at the prospect of sleeping with someone new. For instance, after becoming widowed, many women—and men—feel they would be betraying their late spouse by becoming involved emotionally or physically with someone else.

That's why you probably shouldn't start dating until you've been widowed (or divorced) at least a year, to give you a chance to come to grips with the loss and the ability to get on with your life. Also, you may not want to date a person who hasn't been divorced or widowed for a similar amount of time at least.

Not to throw a bucket of cold water on the subject of sex, but another factor that may dampen desire is fear of contracting sexually transmitted diseases (STDs), including the AIDS virus. The National Institute of

Health estimates that the number of older people with HIV/AIDS is rising—about 10% of all Americans diagnosed with it are 50 years old or older. That translates into 75,000 people. Actually, that number may be much higher, as older people don't often have themselves tested regularly.

Here are some danger signs that this problem will spread even more among this population:

• Older people know less than younger folk about the disease and how it's spread.

• Many health-care workers and educators, unaware that older people can and are contracting the virus, tend to neglect talking to older people about education, testing and prevention.

• Older people are more likely than younger people to write off HIV/AIDS symptoms as normal aches and pains of getting on in years.

• The lack of early detection and treatment means infected elderly people are likely to die sooner than their younger counterparts.

The Mind is Willing, But the Flesh Won't Cooperate

Many physical symptoms may get in the way of sexual desire and performance. Among the most common *for both men and women*:

• Both genders experience reduced levels of testosterone, which drives libido. From ages 20 to 45, testosterone drops sharply in women, according to Dr. John Morley, director of geriatric medicine at St. Louis University. Testosterone gradually begins to wane in men between 40 and 50, and by age 70, most men's testes are no longer producing sufficient amounts.

The timing of when testosterone drops in men and women might explain why their sexual desire at the same age differs so much. An AARP study found that 57% of men 45 and older feel sexual desire at least two or three times a week, while only 22% of women that age did.

- Medications such as some antidepressants can also reduce libido or sexual functioning. If you are taking these medicines, it is worthwhile to share such side effects with your doctor, who may be able to adjust the dosage or switch to another pill that would reduce or remove this side effect.

For women: By 2020 there will be more menopausal than childbearing women. A Harris Interactive study found that, on average, nearly half of menopausal patients experience a loss of sexual desire or a decrease in sexual satisfaction due to menopause. A National Health and Social Life Survey reported that of women age 40 to 59, 21% had difficulty lubricating, 16% said sex wasn't enjoyable, and 10% had pain during sex.

Estrogen can relieve many symptoms, from hot flashes to vaginal dryness. But hormone replacement therapy can exacerbate the lack of testosterone in women. Estrogen increases the substance that holds testosterone in your blood, preventing it from getting to your body.

Women who (rightfully) worry about STDs can kill two birds with one stone—protect themselves from disease and obtain extra lubrication by insisting that their partners use lubricated condoms.

For men: The same National Health and Social Life study found that on average, 16% of men age 40 to 59 were unable to keep an erection and had anxiety about their performance. For many, Viagra has been a blessing. Obviously, it's not for everyone, especially men with heart problems, or those who take nitrates, as the combination can cause dangerously low blood pressure, says the Food and Drug Administration (FDA).

Most men can tolerate Viagra fairly well. The FDA says side effects generally are mild and temporary, and may include headache, flushing, upset stomach, congestion, urinary tract infection, diarrhea and, oddly, visual changes in blue/green colors or increased sensitivity to light.

However, Viagra may not work quite right for everyone. The following interview describes several useful approaches that one couple—Sonya, a 61-year-old woman and Hal, 64—experienced.

After 30-plus years of marriage and an active sex life, Hal became extremely depressed when he began having difficulty getting an erection. He tried Viagra, and it worked—it did what it was supposed to do. But neither of them felt comfortable using it. Viagra didn't improve his libido, which was also flagging. Sonya explains that a Viagra-induced erection "felt unnatural without there being any real desire from him. But I wasn't going to take that as the final way we were going to get through our lives together, without any libido on his part. That was the worst part of it, not that he couldn't get an erection but that he had no desire."

One doctor correctly suspected the problem was extremely low testosterone. A battery of medical tests revealed a benign tumor on Hal's pituitary gland, which regulates the production, among other things, of testosterone. Apparently, this is quite common and quite easy to remedy nonsurgically. There are many forms of supplements—oral, injections and creams. Hal tried them all. Sonya learned to give him the shots, which enormously improved Hal's libido. Later another doctor prescribed a topical cream they both prefer. Sonya adds, "He doesn't get a really strong erection, but he does get enough to make it fun for him as well as for me."

She also says Dr. Saul Rosenthal's book, *Sex Over 40*, helped the couple accept that it was normal to feel a different kind of sexual urgency as they age. "Neither of us were going to reach orgasm as quickly. Hal wouldn't get hard as quickly, and he would lose it and get it back. The book recommended taking a different approach to making love, and encouraged us to experiment with different things instead of just trying to stick it in when it wasn't really hard enough and I wasn't really wet enough." Changing their expectations and opening themselves up to experimenting with new sexual approaches has proved to be liberating, satisfying and fun for both of them.

More recently, Hal, with his libido greatly improved, decided to experiment once again with Viagra. Every once in a while, says Sonya, "he takes a pill and he does enjoy having that large, enormous thing. It takes a little longer for him to climax, which doesn't bother him in the least. Though sometimes I get a little tired!"

Striking the Right Balance

Pardon the pun, but there is a downside to Viagra for some people. With sexual function restored, some men acquire the desire to have sex much more often than their partners. Such women may not welcome their man's reawakened ardor. That can wreak havoc on the marriage and result in infidelity. Even some women who welcomed their husband's renewed abilities found their husbands went knocking on the doors of other, usually much younger, women. These men may have stayed married only because of their inability to perform with other women. They may leave once their doctor scribbles out a prescription.

Men who compensated for their former inability to have intercourse became much more attentive, sensitive lovers. They also acquired more of a taste for "outercourse"—cuddling, massage, masturbation, oral sex and other forms of pleasuring their mates.

And men, too, may find Viagra isn't the end-all, be-all. They may feel disappointed that their ejaculations are not as explosive as in their youth.

Despite all the Internet ads for instant access to this prescription drug, men should discuss the issue, first with their wives, to make sure they are on board. If not, they should consider consulting a marriage therapist to help each partner understand the ramifications of going ahead and not going ahead, and make sure their expectations are realistic. Then, if they decide to give it a whirl, the man should consult his doctor and make sure he is a candidate.

Suddenly Single in the New Dating World

Today, after being married for many years, people can find themselves suddenly single, after a divorce or the death of a spouse. If you find yourself suddenly single, especially if you had been married for several decades to the same person, it can be terrifying to venture into the world of dating. The rules have definitely changed! My primary dating experiences, like the experiences of so many of my peers, go back to the fifties.

It was the era of the blind date, also known as getting "fixed up." The neat thing about it was that the person who arranged the blind date knew something about the people they were bringing together.

Before you went out, you were aware of some things you had in common, such as religion, major interests, type of work, level of education. There was a certain comfort level in the fact that a friend or relative knew and approved of your prospective date.

Until recently, few articles have focused on the dating habits of those 60+. This was because it was thought dating among the elderly was infrequent. Researchers assumed the low rate of remarriage among seniors meant they were not seeking each other out at all romantically.

A fascinating new study by Richard and Kris Bulcroft, "The Nature and Functions of Dating in Later Life," found that older people are just as romantic and are just as interested in having sex as younger couples. They want a long-lasting and intimate personal relationship that will serve as a sexual outlet, and even more importantly, a hedge against loneliness.

Loneliness is a pervasive problem among the elderly. Almost 10 million seniors (about 31% of all non-institutionalized older people) lived alone in 1998.[3]

In 1999, 77% of men 65 and older were married, compared with 43 percent of women in that age group.[4] Among those unmarried, there were 8.4 million widowers and 1.9 million widows, while 2.2 million seniors—8%—were divorced or separated. That may be a small percentage, but it's up from 1.5 million in 1990.

Many seniors are looking for a companion, but they prefer to "go steady," over taking marriage vows.

For many, entering the 21st century dating world is easier desired than done.

Of course, some seniors begin their search in a comfortable venue such as their church or synagogue, or asking friends to fix them up. Personal ads have been around for more than 50 years. Other tried-and-true ways of meeting new love interests include attending high school and college reunions and traveling on senior single tours.

Today there are exciting new ways for older adults to meet potential dating partners:

• **The Internet**, for instance, has become an astonishing global way for people to meet and interact. Many web sites cater especially to older Americans, such as SeniorNet.org and numerous bulletin boards where people with special interests or hobbies can contact each other.

• **Then there are the dating sites.** Would you believe there are more than 900 of them—www.match.com, www.lavalife.com and www.yahoo.com are three of the largest ones. Some are free, but that means anyone can browse the personals. The sites that only allow access to members charge a fee, often ranging from $20 for one month to $99 for a full year. Often it's free to post a profile by filling out a form that allows you to describe yourself: including age, education, job, physical traits, favorite activities, what you're looking for in a date or mate, etc.

You can search the service for people who meet your criteria, but you cannot contact them without paying up. Potential dates can read your profile and have the system generate an e-mail to you without revealing your e-mail address. But with most services, you cannot contact dates unless you sign up as a paid member.

Many people assume these sites attract a higher quality person, on the assumption that people who are willing to pay a fee are more serious about finding that special person.

Many online services focus on members of a particular religious persuasion or professional, age or geographic category.

These online dating sites have become big business, generating more than $300 million in 2002, up from $72 million in 2001. Obviously, the stigma of personal ads—in newspapers, online or via video dating services—has decreased as singles of all ages and backgrounds realize they're not just for losers. They can be a very effective way to target people with characteristics you value.

An excellent book that explains what cyber-dating is all about is *The Online Dating Survival Guide* (E-Solutions Press, 2004), by Dr. Karen Adams and Kate Crenshaw. They evaluate the pros and cons of many of the major dating web sites.

After I was divorced and I was starting to date, my best girlfriend gave me this advice: "If a guy moves in with you, he'll come with his clothes in a plastic bag—just remember to save that bag so he can have it on the way out." My eyes went so wide when she told me that. I had assumed that living with someone implied the relationship was pretty stable and would last. My friend has become fairly cynical on that score, and I suppose I've become a bit more cynical, too.

One mistake I made was dating too soon after my divorce. I only waited about six months before I became involved with someone and yes, he moved in. That relationship lasted a dozen years and ended badly. I think I would have grown and given myself time to heal from my divorce if I had been secure and confident enough to live on my own—for the first time in my life. I had gone from living in my mother's home to marrying at age 18.

I was so terrified of living alone and the loneliness that represented to me, that I didn't take time to get to know that first boyfriend well enough. But you never know where you will meet a new love. I met the current love in my life when I welcomed a new neighbor with a plant. It turns out he was a bachelor and the rest is romantic history.

First Date Survival Tips

Once people have made initial contact through one of the many dating vehicles, they should learn more about each other. E-mail is a popular way to do this. For safety reasons, you should get an extra e-mail address just for this purpose (you can get free e-mail at yahoo.com or hotmail.com), to protect your main personal e-mail address. That way, if you encounter someone who harasses you in any way, you can cancel that address without having to notify your entire social, family and professional network of a changed main address.

Here are a few general tips for dealing with dating online.

- Watch out for someone who seems too perfect.

- Your antenna should go up if someone keeps coming up with excuses for not sending you a photo or giving you a phone number.

- Don't meet someone new until you are really comfortable.

- If your gut instincts tell you to hesitate, listen to them.

- When you do finally make a date, arrange to meet in a well-lit public place and get there in your own car. You might even ask a friend to be there, at a separate corner, as a secret chaperone to intervene if you give them a pre-arranged signal. Or ask a friend to call your cell phone at a pre-arranged time during your date and have a code-word to indicate there is a problem.

If you've gone out, like him or her, but still have questions before your relationship becomes more involved, you can do a criminal, marital, and civil background check (use search keywords "background checks") at many web sites—for a nominal fee. You can also run a "Google" on your prospective date—new lingo that means typing his or her name into a search engine to find out more about the person's professional, community and other personal involvements. Not everyone will have dozens or hundreds of "hits," but you may just find some interesting information.

Okay, you are on your way to meet the person whose voice you've heard over the phone or with whom you have corresponded by e-mail. It's been a long time since you dated. What advice do the dating services give their clients?

First, people form a lasting impression of each other in the first eight to 10 seconds. What your mother told you was right. Stand up straight, dress your best and don't talk about your last relationship—a mistake so many seniors make.

Most of all, let yourself relax, be real and have fun!

Other Resources:

• *50+ and Looking for Love Online*, by Barbara Harrison (Crossing Press, 2000).

• *Funny I Don't Feel Old: How to Flourish After 50*, by Carter Henderson (ICS Press), 1997.

• *The Online Dating Survival Guide*, by Dr. Karen Adams and Kate Crenshaw (E-Solutions Press, 2004).

• *Seasons of the Heart: Men and Women Talk about Love, Sex and Romance after 60*, by Zenith Henkin Gross (New World Library, 2000).

• *Sex over 40*, by Dr. Saul Rosenthal (Jeremy P. Tarcher, 2000).

• *Still Doing It: Women & Men over 60 Write About Their Sexuality*, by Joani Blank (Down There Press, 2000).

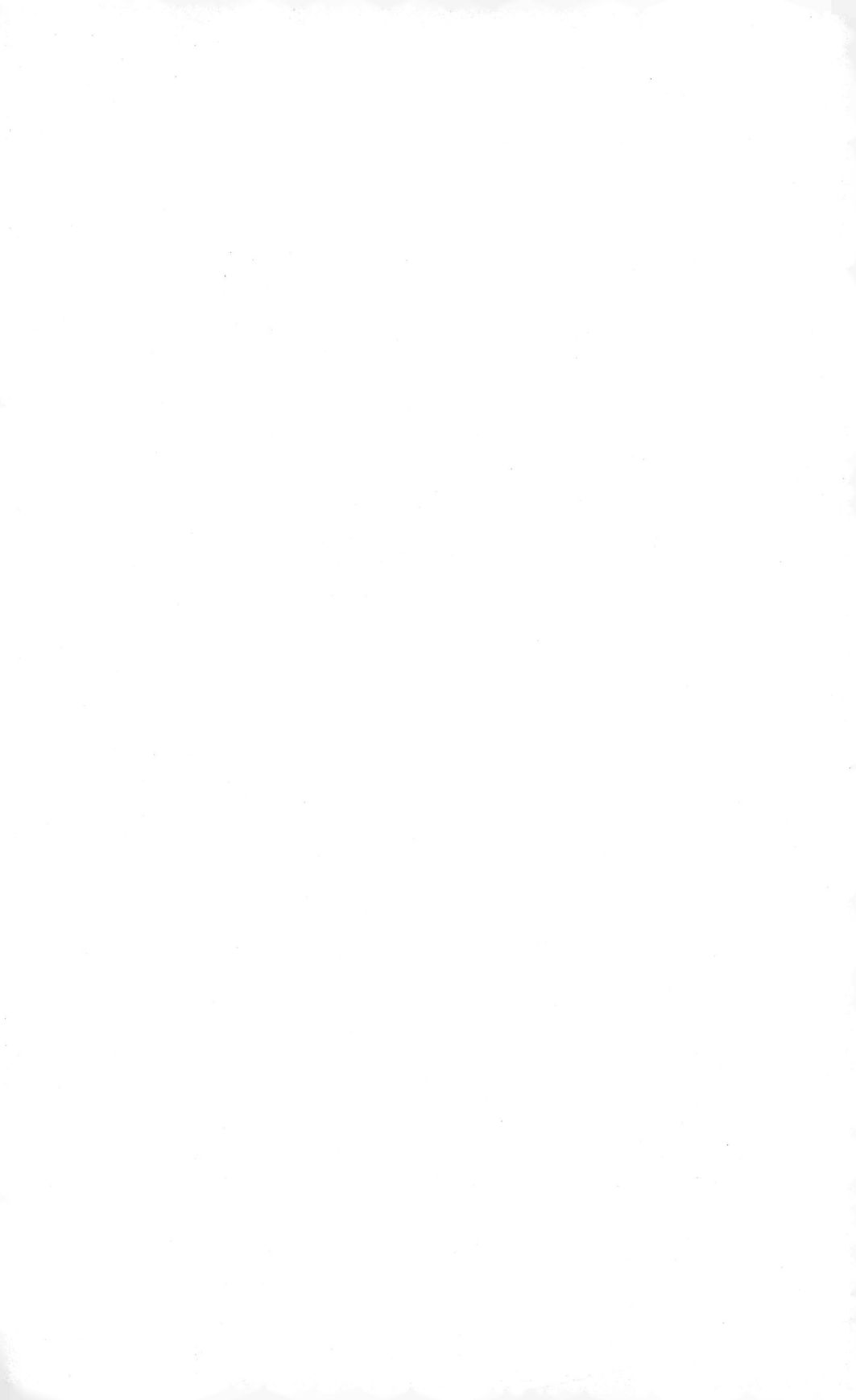

Chapter 6:

DO Try This at Home

Whether you are a 40- or 50-something boomer or a 70-something senior, you may have one or both elderly parents who need your help in their home. Or you might need help living independently in your own home.

Even perfectly healthy aging people may feel emotionally needy or depressed as they realize they are no longer able to live as independently and as they lose friends (or their spouse).

When one's health is increasingly failing, it is difficult to figure out how to adapt the home to accommodate any disabilities, find home-health aides or find another living situation, be it assisted living or a nursing home. Then there's the physical move and all that entails: the sorting through decades of belongings, packing, unpacking and getting settled into a new environment. Of course, you will need to monitor the situation to make sure all evolving needs are met.

In any case, the growing needs of your parents and your own changing needs are likely to tax your time, energy, emotions and possibly finances, as you are called upon to help them adjust or adjust yourself to their new circumstances.

This chapter will walk you through some of the most pressing issues and decisions you may confront, and provide many resources that can offer information and help.

Helping Parents in Their Home

Who wants to leave their home? Not most seniors, according to a recent AARP study, which found that 83% of older Americans want to remain in their current home for their remaining years. They likely feel comfortable and safe there, have nearby friends and perhaps a support network, and enjoy feeling independent. But no matter how comfy, their homes may not meet their needs in later years.

Some modifications may be in order. AARP provides a checklist to test whether a home meets the needs of its aging owner, which you can find on its website (http://www.aarp.org/universalhome/checklist.html). For instance, windows, faucets, doors, locks, drawers and cabinets should all be easy to open and shut. For those in wheelchairs, doors, hallways and bathrooms must be wide enough to navigate. The site also describes possible problems with floors, electric outlets, stairs, appliances, closets, lighting and ventilation and suggests safety and comfort improvements, such as:

- No scatter rugs.

- Handrails on both sides of staircases and outside steps.

- Electric outlets 27 inches above floor.

- Peephole or view panel in front door.

- Walk-in shower with grab bars and portable or adjustable shower seat.

- Hand-held adjustable shower head.

- Non-skid surface for bathtub and shower floor.

- Grab bars by the toilet and tub.

- Bathroom telephone that is reachable if you should fall.

- Adjustable countertops or lower counter for work space in kitchen.

- Rounded kitchen counter tops.

- Sliding shelves in cupboards, lazy susan in corner cabinet.

- First floor bedroom and bath to allow living entirely on one level if necessary.

In addition to modifying the physical space, you may need to make sure that elderly parents have the help they may need with transportation, shopping, cleaning or cooking.

Driving Forces

Speaking of transportation, while many seniors don't drive, they account for 18% of all traffic fatalities. The tragedy in July 2003 in Santa Monica, where an 86-year-old man lost control of his car and killed 10 people and injured dozens more, is an unfortunate example. Those numbers are bound to rise significantly, as the senior population continues to increase. By 2030, more than 32 million drivers over age 75 will still be behind the wheel.[1]

Driving requires split-second decision-making, fast reflexes and good vision and hearing. A decline in one or more of these abilities, which often accompanies aging, will increase the risk of traffic accidents. So will taking some prescription drugs, which can cause side effects such as drowsiness.

There may come a time when you will perceive your elderly parents behind the wheel as a menace to themselves or others. And it might not be terribly easy to convince them of that. You might at least strongly suggest they drive shorter distances, not drive at night, avoid rush hour, stay off major highways and not drive during inclement weather.

You may be able to convince them to take a refresher driver's ed course designed especially for seniors. Thirty-four states and the District of Columbia require discounts in insurance premiums or reductions in infraction points for older people who take the AARP 55 Alive/Mature Driving Program (888-227-7669 or www.aarp.org/55alive). If you are over 55, you might offer to take the course with them!

Some 19 states have special provisions for the renewal of driving licenses for seniors, which include some combination of knowledge tests, vision and road tests. Contact your State Department (or Registry) of Motor Vehicles to find out the age-testing requirements in your state.

Such testing is a great idea, but let's not forget that a person's ability should never be based on age alone. A good driver can be 18 or 80. So can a bad driver.

Some cars, such as the Lincoln Town Car, are safer and more senior friendly. For instance, the Town Car has an extra set of radio and temperature controls on the steering wheel to keep maximum attention on the road. Cadillacs come with infrared night vision technology to make night driving easier. Some automakers are redesigning door handles and gearshifts that are easier for arthritis sufferers to use, and easier-to-read instrument panels. Airbags are still a hazard for older people, whose fragile bones might break on inflation.

The capacity to go from one place to another is vital to seniors' sense of well-being. After they stop driving, their need to get around does not simultaneously come to a screeching halt. Special vans in many states provide rides for seniors. However, they are usually restricted to visits to doctors' offices, hospitals, senior centers and adult day-care centers. Some senior centers use their vans for group shopping trips or special events.

Unfortunately, many seniors assume this driving service is just for the poor. Some are too embarrassed to take these vans. While many cities provide excellent mass transportation, fewer than 10% of older adults ride public busses or subways. One reason is that 70% of seniors live in suburban or rural locations, where transit is either non-existent or limited. Physically challenged elders may have trouble climbing stairs or boarding a bus, or may fear becoming victims of crime.

Solutions or alternatives exist for most of these limitations. For instance, the National Academy on an Aging Society wants to put low-platform buses in service to attract more seniors.

Other Resources:

National Highway Traffic Safety Administration
www.nhtsa.dot.gov
888-327-4236

Age Lab, Massachusetts Institute of Technology
http://web.mit.edu/agelab

American Automobile Association
www.aaa.com

Federal Transit Administration
www.fta.dot.gov

National Association of State Units on Aging
www.nasua.org

Getting Good Home Care

Studies show that less than 11% of the care comes from a paid home-care worker. In fact, relatives care for four out of five of the disabled elderly in the U.S.

Today, because we're living so much longer, many 70-year-olds are taking care of 90-year-olds. The Long Term Care Campaign says the average woman can expect to spend 17 years caring for a child and 18 years caring for an elderly parent. But caregiving is no longer predominately a women's issue. Men now make up 44% of the caregiver population.

Also, because many baby boomers are not having children until they are in their late thirties or early forties, they may find themselves raising young children and caring for ailing parents at the same time. Family caregivers provide elder care an average of four hours a day, seven days a week.

A recent MetLife "Juggling Act Study"[2] found that:

• Nearly 25% of all households will have at least one adult who provides care for an elderly person at some point during a 12-month period.

• Sixty-four percent of these caregivers are employed, and must juggle their personal and professional responsibilities.

• Caregivers face significant losses in career development, salary and retirement income, and out-of-pocket expenses.

Limited help may be available, thanks to the Family and Medical Leave Act, which requires companies with more than 50 employees to allow employees an unpaid leave of 12 weeks if they have been on the job at least one year. The weeks do not have to be consecutive. While the Family and Medical Leave Act can be used for elder care, it doesn't help with long-term needs.

Spouses make up one of the largest groups of caregivers. The National Family Caregivers Association reports spousal caregivers do not get consistent help from other family members. Its recent study reveals that as many as 75% of spousal caretakers are "going it alone." As a result, 61% of solo care givers experience depression and anxiety; 25% experience stomach disorders. Of the many emotions caregivers feel, guilt is the most pervasive. What's worse, they don't realize that all these emotions are normal given their circumstances.

It is in everyone's best interest to provide the caregiver as much support as possible. That might mean pitching in some care. For instance, if one of your parents is caring for the other parent, you can give the caregiver regular breaks, find other sources of help such as aides, information and services. If the caregiver gets to the point where he or she can no longer take care of the ailing person, you may need to take a more active role yourself. Or, perhaps you are already providing all or some care yourself.

So here are two critical things to consider:

- **Is the caregiver adequately skilled to handle the job?** Most are not, because the job is usually thrust upon them following an emergency health problem with the older person. The Home Care Companion series of videos (1-888-846-7008, http://www.homecarecompanion.com) teaches caregivers how to care for someone who is bedridden, how to help someone in a wheel chair without hurting yourself and other important skills.

- **Where can you find quality support?** Your local Area Agency on Aging can direct you to the new National Family Caregiver Support Program, a federal program that grants money to states to provide information, assistance, training and counseling for caregivers. It also can provide opportunities for caretakers to take a break from their stressful duties.

Other useful federally funded programs are the Senior Volunteer and the Retired Senior Volunteer programs, as well as the Senior Home Companion Volunteer program. These organizations help family caregivers get their errands done, attend a family caregivers' support group, or simply relax.

DO Try This at Home

The Elder Care Locators (800-677-1116) can help long-distance or working relatives find home aides.

Some Useful Books and Organizations Devoted to Caregiving:

Caregiving: The Spiritual Journey of Love, Loss, and Renewal, by Beth Witrogen McLeod (John Wiley & Sons, 2000).

Caring for Yourself While Caring for Your Aging Parents: How to Help, How to Survive, by Claire Berman (Owl Book, 2001).

The Comfort of Home: An Illustrated Step-by-Step Guide for Caregivers, by Maria M. Meyer, et al (CareTrust Publications LLC, 1998).

The Complete Eldercare Planner: Where to Start, Questions to Ask, and How to Find Help, by Joy Loverde (Hyperion, 1997).

The Fearless Caregiver: How to Get the Best Care for Your Loved One and Still Have a Life of Your Own, by Gary Barg (Capital Books Inc., 2001). Mr. Barg also gives seminars and publishes *Today's Caregiver* magazine.
www.caregiver.com
800-829-2734

Keeping Them Healthy, Keeping Them Home, by Ellen M. Caruso, R.N. (Health Information Press, 1998).

Quick Tips for Caregivers, by Marion Karpinski (Healing Arts Communications, 2000).

The Well Spouse Foundation
www.wellspouse.org
A national, not-for-profit membership organization that gives support to wives, husbands and partners of the chronically ill and/or disabled. Support groups meet monthly, share their thoughts and feelings openly with others facing similar circumstances in a supportive, non-judgmental environment, and provide information on practical issues facing spousal caregivers.

Caregiving is a problem that is not likely to go away, with people living longer and hospitals sending patients home earlier, and professional outside care becoming more and more expensive.

Coping with Loneliness

One of the heartbreaks of aging is some degree of loneliness. Facing the physical, emotional, medical and spiritual challenges of aging alone can cause elderly people to feel isolated, scared and depressed. Companionship is critical to health and happiness.

• **Senior centers and/or adult day care.** For family caregivers who must work or who live far away, adult day care is often a wonderful resource. These centers usually provide transportation, supervision, meals as well as some health and medical monitoring. It gives people who participate a wonderful chance to socialize with other older adults.

For instance, the Lenox Hill Senior Center at St. Peter's Church in Manhattan offers classes in yoga, which has members who can still stand on their heads, reports the *The New York Times*.[3] A business group for members not ready for full retirement has members brainstorming and sharing access to their professional network. There are also foreign language classes. But members nixed a bereavement group and no one showed when a doctor came to discuss cancer.

Some seniors, though, resist going because they have an image that senior centers are depressing places, that they consist of hunched over people playing cards or bingo, complaining about their ailments. Some are, in fact, exactly like that. But a growing number of senior centers, such as Lenox Hill, attract well-educated, energetic and upbeat people who are more active and demand more interesting alternatives.

See if you can find a local senior center that offers meditation or Shakespeare classes instead of bingo and cards. Offer to go with your parent to check out the place together, and help them set up transportation if necessary.

Benefits and Drawbacks of Pets

It's important to find other ways to compensate for seniors' shrinking social circle, as friends and family pass away, as children and grandchildren grow up and move away, and as retirement represents the loss of professional colleagues. One way to combat resulting loneliness is the companionship and affection that pets can bring. Furry, finned or feathered friends can provide many physical, psychological and social benefits, aid relaxation and give a sense of purpose and responsibility that comes with the daily routines involved in caring for a pet. Walking a dog provides exercise and an opportunity to meet and socialize with other pet owners; and their presence at home can provide protection.

In fact, a recent three-year study [4] of more than 5,500 people found that pet owners had lower blood pressure, triglyceride and cholesterol levels than non-pet owners.

However, pet ownership also comes with some drawbacks:

• **Pets can be expensive.** Licenses, training classes, spaying, veterinary care, grooming, toys, food and inoculations can add up quickly. Suggested solution: Sharing a pet with a neighbor will cut those costs in half.

• **Many apartments, assisted living and nursing home facilities don't allow pets.** Make sure you check out such restrictions before bringing an animal home. Suggested solution: "Borrow" a neighbor or friend's pet—offer to walk the pet, or cat- or dog-sit for vacationing friends.

• **Many animals require more care and attention than elderly people are able to handle.** For instance, pets can get fleas, scratch furniture and have "accidents." Some small dogs, such as terriers, are very hyper and require a lot of exercise to stay calm, and they often bark at noise or visitors. Make sure to choose an animal that will fit your lifestyle. Suggested solution: Hire a local teenager whom you can pay to walk the dog when the weather is bad or you're not feeling well, or help you with other pet-related responsibilities you can't handle.

For help adopting a pet, contact your local ASPCA or Petfinder (www.petfinder.org).

Eventually, you may need to make a very difficult decision with, or for, your parents: whether or not they will be safer or need the services of some form of assisted living or a nursing home.

Assisted Living: the Latest Trend in Senior Housing

Assisted living is a relatively new housing concept. The United States began to adopt it in the 1980s, based on a Scandinavian model of senior housing and care. The concept quickly became popular because it offers older Americans an attractive mixture of independence and personal care.

Assisted living complexes are home to 800,000 Americans whose average age is 84. Some of the 10,000-plus facilities in operation today (90% of which were built in the last decade) are stand-alone and some are part of continuing-care retirement communities that offer varying levels of help and medical supervision. They can best be described as a cross between an apartment and hotel, with services for semi-independent elderly and a nursing home for those who need more comprehensive assistance.

Most assisted living facilities include: 24-hour supervision, three meals a day in a group dining room, social and recreational activities, transportation, laundry and housekeeping services. Some also offer (for an extra charge) personal care services such as help with eating, bathing, dressing, and taking medicines. Nearly a quarter of assisted living facilities have special units for older Americans in the early stages of Alzheimers. According to AARP, many larger assisted living complexes offer such amenities as a library, café, beauty parlor, and chapel.

The continuing-care model provides the most options, combining different kinds of services in a single setting. You can start out living independently, and when your needs become greater, you can switch to assisted living and then to a nursing home located right on the property. This guaranteed care as you age comes at a high price, of course. Continuing care residences usually require an entry fee as well as monthly fees from $1,500 to $5,000.

According to Consumer Reports' *Complete Guide to Health Services for Seniors*, prices vary greatly, but on average cost $2,000 in monthly rent and fees. Rate increases can average 5% to 7% annually.

The most commonly asked question is who pays for assisted living's monthly rent and fees? Not Medicare, which only provides short-term acute care for the elderly. Ninety-five percent of residents must pay for these services out of their own pocket, although some people have long-term insurance that may partly cover assisted living. Government payments have been extremely limited. Presently, 37 states use the Medicaid home and community-based waiver programs to help finance some assisted-living services.

Assisted living facilities are not substitutes for nursing homes. With the exception of more expensive continuing-care communities, about 36% of all residents eventually go to nursing homes because the assisted-living facility cannot accommodate their increasing needs. An additional 2% go to nursing homes because they have exhausted the means to pay for assisted living. Unfortunately, some seniors use the entire pool of their long-term care insurance proceeds on assisted living and have nothing left when the time comes for nursing home care.

While assisted living facilities are very popular and have experienced phenomenal growth, they are not without serious problems. The main one is that, unlike nursing homes, the federal government does not regulate assisted living communities; states do. The result: widely varying standards relating to such things as the number and training of staff, fire and safety regulations.

What you don't know may hurt you. Most residents enter an assisted living facility expecting to live there forever. But buried in the fine print, the contract they signed stipulates that physical or mental decline can be grounds for discharge. Facilities in many states can evict residents with little notice. Another unpleasant surprise for many assisted living residents are hidden fees for things they thought were already paid for. In fact, elder law attorney and *A Touch of Grey* co-host Stephen J.J. Weisman of Cambridge, Massachusetts points out that Congress recently held hearings to consider regulating the assisted living industry. "There is no consistency from state to state, even about the definition," he points out. Weisman cautions consumers to beware of the following clauses:

• **Refunds.** Can a person get a partial or total refund if the agreement is terminated? Some facilities will fully refund entrance fees, which can be substantial; some will not, even if a resident must leave to obtain greater care.

• **Fee increases.** What kind of provisions does the contract have if the residents can't afford increases in fees? This is a big issue. Sometimes there are provisions for reduced fees if residents don't use certain services temporarily—for instance, if they're going on vacation, or hospitalized, does the facility still hold residents responsible for meals and other services?

• **Changing terms.** Can the facility change the terms of the agreement while a resident is there? Most agreements allow them to make changes.

• **Grounds for eviction.** What are they, and does the contract specify any kind of right of appeal?

The best guidelines I found for checking into an assisted living facility came from The Consumer Consortium on Assisted Living:

• Carefully assess your physical, financial, mental and life-style needs. Remember: assisted living is not for those who don't like living and eating in a group setting.

• Visit as many facilities as you can.

• Narrow your choices down to two or three, return to these facilities and ask a lot of questions. Eat a meal there. Stop by several times, unannounced, near meal times, or early evening to see how the facility is managed at busy and low-staff times.

• Ask to see the resident agreement. The contract should show fees, services provided, facility and resident responsibilities and much more.

• Be sure to consult with an attorney, preferably an elder specialist, before signing anything.

DO Try This at Home

- Review the licensing or certification report.

- Call the long-term ombudsman and find out if there are any complaints. To find a local ombudsman call 800-677-1116.

It's important to consider future housing options well before they are needed. Waiting until health problems or disabilities set in may disqualify one from entry!

For More Information:

Consumer Reports' *Complete Guide to Health Services for Seniors*, by Trudy Lieberman and the Editors of *Consumer Reports*.

American Association of Homes and Services for the Aging
(800) 5089422
www.aahsa.org

Assisted Living Federation of America
(703) 691-8100
www.alfa.org

What to Look for in a Nursing Home

Few people want to look for a nursing home for a loved one. Unfortunately, at some point such a facility may be the only safe and feasible option. While only 4% of America's seniors currently live in a nursing home, those who do have a wider range of options today based on each resident's needs.

For instance, most nursing homes today offer rehabilitative care that developed in response to the present policy of hospitals releasing patients quicker and sicker. Rehab units help patients return to as high a level of functioning as possible in the shortest period of time, so patients can return to living in their own home. Services are provided by licensed occupational and physical therapists, as well as registered nurses and licensed practical nurses.

With the ability to replace even more of our worn-out body parts, people will likely check into rehab units a number of times during their lifetime.

Nursing homes in the 21st century have evolved into what are now called skilled-care facilities. A skilled-care facility, in addition to offering rehabilitative care, often also offers special care such as IV therapy, wound management and breathing support with ventilators. Other special-care units deal with behavioral problems that stem from dementia. They usually provide security to keep residents from wandering, have high staff-patient ratios, and provide comprehensive programming designed for confused and disoriented patients.

A skilled-care facility can also provide long-term care, including nursing supervision, but it is primarily focused on custodial care. The average age of a nursing home resident is 84. Services are aimed at keeping the person safe and healthy, but not at improving his or her condition. When many people think of nursing homes, they think of them as a place for someone whose physical or mental condition requires permanent, round-the-clock care. Unfortunately, Medicare rarely covers this kind of custodial care. Medicaid, a federal-state administered welfare program, will cover these long-term care costs, but only after a nursing home resident has spent down his or her financial assets.

To find out what's available in your community, the Eldercare Locator (800-677-1116) is the place to call for help getting in touch with your local agency on aging, which can supply you with a list of nursing homes in your area. Be sure to ask whether the facility is for profit or not-for-profit. There are only a handful of not-for-profit nursing homes. They generally have higher staff-patient ratios. Your family doctor, local social worker or the recommendation of a friend who has a family member in a nearby long-term care facility are other good sources of referrals.

Selecting a particular nursing home can be difficult. Trudy Lieberman in Consumers Reports' *Complete Guide to Health Services for Seniors* gives some great advice on what your main concerns should be:

• The staff-to-patient ratio on all shifts.

• The attentiveness and qualifications of the staff.

- Pleasant and safe environment. Nursing home should be attractive, bright, clean and odor free.

- Provisions for privacy and protection of personal property.

- Meal quality.

- Meaningful activities for residents.

To find out the quality of care at a particular nursing home, ask for the facility's state inspection form 2567. States, usually through their health department, are responsible for carrying out and enforcing federal regulations that apply to nursing homes. State surveyors make unannounced visits every nine to 15 months to check on the quality of patient care, as well as the enforcement of safety rules. Areas of strength and weakness are noted, as are any deficiencies. The state inspection report is supposed to be prominently displayed in every health care facility. Ask to see it and take the time to read it.

Another excellent source of information about a nursing home you are considering is your state's long-term care ombudsman. In 1978, the ombudsman program was established across the country as part of the Older Americans Act. The ombudsmen know the good, the bad and the ugly about the nursing homes in their jurisdiction. They resolve complaints on behalf of nursing home patients and make periodic visits to nursing homes when there are problems. To talk to an ombudsman, contact your Area Agency on Aging or your state's Office of the Aging.

The government also has recently released data that will make it easier for consumers to judge the quality of care in 17,000 nursing homes. For each long-term care facility, the government published 10 measures of performance and quality, such as the percentage of residents who were in physical restraints, or had bedsores, pain, or symptoms of acute confusion or delirium.

You should ask yourself two intangible questions when thinking about a nursing home for a loved one: Does it seem like a friendly place? Would I want to live here?

Further Resources:

Medicare
www.Medicare.gov
800-MEDICARE (800-633-4227)
Click the section called "Nursing Home Compare" for information on the government's report card on nursing homes.

When Someone You Love Needs Nursing Home, Assisted Living, or In-Home Care, by Robert F. Bornstein, Ph.D. and Mary A. Languirand, Ph.D. (W.W. Norton & Company, 2002)

As Parents Age, by Joseph A. Ilardo, Ph.D. (Vanderwyke & Burnham, 1998)

Consumer Reports' *Complete Guide to Health Services for Seniors,* by Trudy Lieberman & the Editors of *Consumer Reports*

Making the Move

A growing number of adult children feel anxious when their parents' are about to move. What is their role? How can they help? Where should they start? "Particularly if the seniors are moving from a long-occupied family home with many memory-laden possessions, a lot needs to be worked out," says Amherst, Masschusetts-based Barbara Perman, founder of Moving Mentor, which helps families plan and execute a move.

With a background in education and psychology, Perman understands the feelings that come up for both generations when the family home will be sold. "Some people become sad, angry, scared, drained, confused, exhausted, overwhelmed, paralyzed," says Perman. "After acknowledging these feelings, my task is to help them see the move as an opportunity — a chance to reflect on the past and to enter the threshold of a new and fulfilling phase of life. I make a strong distinction between merely moving (relocating one's stuff) and 'moving on' — making a healthy transition into a new phase of life."

Perman has many ideas for making the process as stress-free as possible. Here are just a few of her suggestions:

- **If you wait until you're ready, it's already too late!** Leave a minimum of three months to a year to put things in order, make thoughtful decisions, and move in a healthy way. It takes time to move in a healthy way, to become educated about options and make a good choice about where to move, and then to sift through a lifetime of belongings and decide what is going and what will be left behind.

- **Allow time to grieve.** Perman points out that the American Psychological Association lists moving among the 10 most stressful experiences in life! Taking pictures of every room to make a memory book can help remind the person of happy times without holding on to the growing burden of the family homestead.

- **Sort and disperse possessions** into three categories: definitely keep, definitely don't need and undecided. You can do this physically by using bags or boxes and/or visually by using removable stickers in assorted colors to designate your categories. Perman emphasizes that cleaning out makes room for new life.

You can find more tips from Perman, plus information about her *Moving Workbook & Planning Guide*, video, audiotape and other resources at www.movingmentor.com.

Keeping Tabs

Wherever you or your aging parents live, it's important to make sure that they are safe. That includes finding a way to check that any housemates or caregivers are treating them with dignity and not abusing or neglecting them in any way.

Every year an estimated 2.1 million older American adults are victims of physical, psychological or other forms of abuse and neglect, including financial exploitation. The American Psychological Association believes that for every elder abuse case that is reported there are five that not have been reported.

Most such abuse occurs right in the home. In fact, children are the most frequent abusers of the elderly. Spouses, other family members and caregivers are ranked as the next most likely abusers of the elderly. While the perpetrators are as likely to be women as men, the majority of victims are women.

The National Academy of Aging believes that in some cases, elder abuse is simply a continuation of abuse that has been occurring in the family for many years. If a woman has been continually abused by her husband, she is not likely to report abuse when she is very old and in poor health. On the other hand, a woman who has been abused for years may turn her rage on her husband when his health fails. Also, adult children who experienced violence growing up may turn the tables on their abusive parents when they become disabled and withhold needed care.

Family stress can often trigger elder abuse. When a frail or disabled older parent moves into a family member's home, the lifestyle adjustments can be overwhelming. In addition, some families find themselves with an additional burden paying for the health care an aging parent needs.

While most nursing home citations in 2001 were relatively minor, one in 10 were for incidents that placed residents at risk of death or serious injury. To prevent elder abuse, Congress—in particular the Senate Aging Committee—has proposed some preventive measures in long-term care facilities such as mandatory criminal checks for all staff members and mandatory reporting by long-term care facilities of suspected elder abuse. Fines for noncompliance could be as high as $100,000.

The public, law enforcement, judges and lawyers need to learn how to spot elder abuse. Bank personnel should be trained to recognize when something is amiss in an elderly person's financial situation. I also believe the government should create a national policy on elder abuse. Right now, each state has different standards about who should be protected and what form that protection should take. A national elder-abuse prosecution system should be modeled after the very successful child-abuse prosecution system.

Other Resources:

The Elder Abuse Center
www.elderabusecenter.org

Your local **Area Agency on Aging**
Check your local yellow pages.
For help with a particular problem in a nursing home, your home or someone else's. Your local agency can refer you to someone in its ombudsman program, and help you locate respite services that can help prevent further abuse and neglect.

Eldercare Locator
800-677-1116
To help relatives or friends who don't live near you.

Chapter 7

Grannies Getting Off Their Fannies:
Rethinking and Redefining Grandparents' Role

My first grandchild, Michael, is already a teenager and driving. Does that make me feel old? No way! If anything, becoming a grandparent has helped me feel younger than ever—even childlike!

Perhaps this is partly because I know I'm in very good company. According to Global Starch Worldwide, a global marketing research firm, 31% of adults—or about 60 million Americans—are grandparents. By 2010, the government estimates that there will be 80 million U.S. grandparents. The National Survey of American Households indicates the average age of a first-time grandparent is 47, and that the typical grandparent has five grandchildren and, in some cases, great grandchildren (25% of grandparents have great grandchildren!). With people living well into their eighties and nineties, one could very well be a grandparent for nearly half of one's life!

But mostly, I feel energized, not enervated at the reality of being a grandparent because the role of this growing army of grandparents is more important than ever—especially with the explosion in the divorce rate. Grandparents can often be the family glue in today's increasingly mobile, single-parent or blended-family households. Grandparents can be an island of stability amid a turbulent family sea.

Diane Marcus, a University of Cincinnati professor of social work and an expert on aging, says today's grandparents are acting as "the keepers of the family" more than ever before. "They are contributing enormously and derive a lot of pleasure from the family. They provide emotional assistance, tangible support and intangible support. And they are thrilled to be able to do that."[1]

"The state of American grandparenting is strong," agrees Gretchen Straw, associate research director of the AARP Research Group, which recently conducted a national survey of grandparents.[2] "Most grandparents see their grandchildren regularly and connect in a number of ways. The relationship is a rewarding one."

One of the most enthusiastic grandparents I have interviewed is Emmy-award-winning comedian, actor, director and author, Billy Crystal. He was so charmed at the prospect of becoming a grandfather, that he wrote what became a best-selling children's book, *I Already Know I Love You* (HarperCollins, 2004). The idea emerged wen his daughter, Jennifer was five-months pregnant, and he accompanied her to the doctors office for her ultrasound. "It was like an aquarium," Crystal told my *A Touch of Grey* radio audience. "And I just went, 'Hi, I'm waiting for you.' And I thought, what am I waiting to do? And I went home and wrote this book, which is a list of simple things in life about what you're waiting to do with this unborn child." Crystal mentions activities such as taking a nap together and rooting for the Yankees, flying a kite and baiting a hook. While the rhymes are sometimes forced and awkward, his passion is contagious.

After spending the summer with his then 15-month-old granddaughter, Ella, Crystal wrote another book, about her first year of life, called *One Was Fun*, to be published Fathers Day, 2005. Crystal says although he, like many comedians, is a tough audience, Ella "gets belly laughs out of me, just doing the simplest things." And it's those simple things that are most rewarding to him as a grandparent: "That smile between us, that little giggle, that little hand to hold my index finger. That stuff is just so profound to me," he says.

Grandparenting is, for many, an opportunity to make up for some of what they feel they may not have done quite right as parents. Crystal agrees: "It was almost more emotional when Ella was born, than it was when Jenny was born in some ways, because it comes at a certain time in your life where time becomes more precious." In my case, I married early and became a stay-at-home mom, juggling the typical (of my generation) responsibilities of taking care of the house, my husband and four children.

After I divorced when I was in my forties, I first earned a college degree and forged a career that led to my becoming the CEO of Focus Communications, a media company that—as I explain in earlier chapters—owns a radio network, *TALKERS* magazine (the leading trade magazine for talk radio and television) and Talk Radio News Service, a Washington, D.C.-based news bureau. I also host the nationally syndicated radio show *A Touch of Grey*.

As much fulfillment as my professional, personal and charitable endeavors bring me, becoming a grandmother has truly liberated my "inner child." I was too trapped in an unhappy marriage to feel young at heart while I was raising my four children: Neal (now an elder law attorney); Ellen (a therapist and mother of Michael, Heather and Daniel); Paul (a lawyer for the state of Connecticut and father of Josh, Anna and Emily); and Mark (a financial planner who recently married).

Now that some of my children have their own children, I am thrilled to watch (and help) my grandkids grow, and I have more energy, time and money to lavish on Michael, Heather, Daniel, Josh, Anna and Emily than I was able to devote to my children.

Last year, for example, I had a wonderful time shopping for my grandchildren's holiday presents. I found a blue stuffed unicorn for little Anna, which sings a song when you squeeze its horn. After I brought the gifts home and was about to wrap them, I was so enraptured with the unicorn that I couldn't resist keeping it for myself! (Of course, I went right back to the store to buy another one for her.) Now we can play with our unicorns together!

I also love trains, probably as a result of taking weekly trips when I was a child with my own grandmother to New York City by train, for my asthma shots. My grandmother, Florence Korn Lehman, is my role model for what a loving grandparent can and should be. Despite her petite 5'2" frame, she had considerable energy. She devoted a great deal of that energy to doting on me and my brother. Whether it was fussing over an elaborate costume to ensure I'd win a costume contest (I did!) or regaling us with exciting stories that she would make up spontaneously to make long trips pass more quickly, she always made me feel I was terribly important.

But let's face it, times have changed. As loving, attentive and generous as she was, my grandmother seemed so old to me! I can't imagine her having, let alone playing with, her own set of toy trains, as I do (a treasured gift from my significant other, Jay) or sitting on the floor for a tea party.

Today's grandparents, like Billy Crystal, who is in his mid-fifties, are much more youthful, energetic and "with it." Professor Marcus explains, "I don't think that the level of grandparents' commitment has changed, and I don't think grandparents love their grandchildren more now than they used to, but they do have many more years of free time. Very often when people retire today, they still feel strong and able, and so they can do more than they used to." She also points out that family size is smaller and grandparents have fewer grandchildren vying for their attention.

"We tend to think of grandparents as old folks with false teeth and gray hair, sitting in rocking chairs. The age of 47 today is not what 47 was a couple of generations ago," says Margaret Hollidge, senior program coordinator for AARP. "We're healthier, more active and better educated." Many dress stylishly, exercise regularly and travel far and wide to exotic places. That's a far cry from the stereotypical grandma with a babushka, slaving in a hot kitchen or a sedentary gramps slouched in an easy chair with a pipe and the newspaper.

It would simply never have occurred to me when I was a little girl, to ask my grandmother to play dolls or fly a kite with me, as I love to do with my grandkids. Yet many are not taking advantage of a world of opportunities to plan creative activities with their grandchildren.

AARP's survey identified the top five activities grandparents engage in with their grandchildren:

- Eating together (either in or out).

- Watching a TV comedy.

- Staying overnight.

- Shopping for clothes.

- Engaging in exercise/sports.

Forty-three percent of grandparents surveyed by AARP say it is "very easy" to come up with potential activities for a grandchild, and another 25% say it is "somewhat easy." Those who feel clueless about finding creative ways to interact with their grandchildren should consider that the single most important thing they can do is build shared and treasured memories together. Activities can be simple and inexpensive: cooking, making a craft together or simply reading together. Below we will mention other meaningful and creative activities.

Grannies Getting Off Their Fannies 79

You also may benefit from a growing number of grandparenting classes. Many hospitals, for instance, hold sessions for expecting grandparents. Among other things, they teach practical skills such as proper use of car seats, the latest information on nutrition, infant sleeping patterns and the psychology of rearing happy and healthy children.

Of grandparents who are not caregivers and who do not live in the same household as grandchildren, 44% see a grandchild every week. Another 25% see a grandchild at least once a month. Almost a third of grandparents (31%) both see and speak by phone to a grandchild each week. Slightly more than one in 10 grandparents (12%) have little contact with a grandchild, seeing or talking on the phone with them every few months or less. In this chapter we will talk about some of the countless creative ways to interact with grandchildren today:

• Traveling with grandkids.

• Volunteering together.

• Communicating with grandkids.

• Transmitting the family history, lore and values.

Yet grandparenting today also brings many new challenges, which we will also explore:

• Redefining your self-image and role as a grandparent.

• Spoiling the grandkids.

• Raising grandchildren. Decreased family stability has resulted in a record number of grandparents assuming the role of primary caregiver.

Traveling with Your Grandkids

Some grandparents are choosing to bond with a grandchild or grandchildren by taking them on a trip. Many tour operators, realizing the value of the grandparent market, now offer intergenerational packages. Helena Koenig, who founded Grandtravel® in 1987 (www.grandtrvl.com, 800-247-7651), says the most common destination is a safari in Kenya, followed by London, Paris, parks in western U.S. and Alaska. A grandmother of nine herself, Koenig considers grandparents and their grandchildren to be ideal travel partners. "Many grandparents are widowed, and the companionship of their grandchildren is indication they will live forever," she explains. "And they enjoy each other's company. We've never sent anyone home for homesickness or bad behavior."

Trips can range from intergenerational camps with outdoor activities to cruises with activities for children of all ages.

Keep in mind that you don't need deep pockets to take your grandchildren on a vacation. You can spend a weekend or even day trip at a nearby village or town, a local museum or show, the beach, or get tickets for a wonderful train trip to a city one-to-three hours away, like my grandmother took me on. If you're in shape, take (or rent) bicycles on a nearby bike path.

Volunteering Together

Arrange to spend one Sunday a month (or more) volunteering at some local nursing home, children's hospital, soup kitchen or other meaningful philanthropic activity. You are bound to share many bonding moments as well as teach them how good it feels to contribute to other people's needs, not just their own. You can help them experience pride and joy that comes from giving of themselves.

One study found that 43% of people age 75 and older said they volunteer. Seniors have the time, talent and experience to share with others. Getting a grandchild involved is a double good deed!

Not sure how to find a volunteer activity you can perform with your grandkids? Senior Corps, administered by the Corporation for National and Community Service, now offers an online volunteer recruitment system that has a database of more than 50,000 volunteer activities for people 55 and older at www.seniorcorps.org. Users simply plug in their ZIP code, how far they're willing to travel, and what sorts of causes or services they want to become involved with, such as youth/children, disabilities, health, hunger, eldercare or homelessness. The system provides a list of available opportunities with short descriptions. Users then choose the activity that interests them and can contact the organization.

For grandparents who have difficulty getting around, another option is for you and your grandchildren to become online volunteers. VolunteerMatch's web site (www.volunteermatch.org/virtual) can match you with nonprofit groups that sponsor services you can perform from the Internet. Two common online volunteer actives are technical assistance (online research, translating material into another language for a nonprofit agency) and direct contact via e-mail or a chat room (such as electronically visiting a homebound person, providing e-mentoring or helping students with homework).

Communicating with Grandkids

Many grandparents are quite computer literate; others are computer-phobic. But more and more grandparents find themselves sitting in front of a video screen playing a game or surfing the net with their grandkids or e-mailing them across the miles. Indeed, computers—and specifically the Internet—will play an ever-larger role in enriching relationships between grandparents and grandchildren, says Steve Barsh, CEO of iGrandparents.com. Americans who are 50 and beyond are the fastest growing segment of first-time online users today, at a time when wide geographic distances commonly separate family members. Barsh says that 40% of people 50 and older have a computer at home compared with 29% in 1996. Americans over 50 spend 47% more time online than the average for all other age groups.

Of course, the good old telephone is an important element of maintaining an open line of communication between you and your grandchildren. In fact, an increasing number of teens and pre-teens have their own cell phones. But e-mail is often easier for both the younger and the older generations to exchange information, photos and artwork. The bonus with teenagers is that they tend to reveal much more of themselves using this form of communication than they do over the phone. If you're on the upper end of the technical continuum, you can even videotape yourself reading a book or record a greeting for a special occasion and e-mail it to them.

Whether you're chatting on the phone or trading online "instant messages," it's not always easy finding topics you will both feel comfortable and interesting to discuss. Dr. Ruth Westheimer, during a recent appearance on my *A Touch of Grey* radio show, suggests ways to communicate from a distance with grandchildren:

• Buy a pre-schooler a camera to take pictures of his or her friends, artwork or family outings. Have their parents send it to you, so you can discuss the photos the next time you speak on the phone. "If you say, 'I saw the picture of your best friend, and how pretty she is,' then there is a conversation."

• For older kids who don't necessarily feel motivated to write letters, you can make and send them self-addressed, stamped postcards with yes-or-no questions they can check off: "Did you get my package?" "Did you like it?" And more open-ended questions such as "What are you doing with it?" The point is to "make it easier to communicate," insists Dr. Ruth, whose book, *Dr. Ruth Talks About Grandparents* (Madison Books, 2001), was recently published.

Transmitting Family History, Lore and Values

I was shocked to learn from the 2002 AARP survey that only 33% of grandparents report talking about family history with their children or grandchildren. This is one area in which you are uniquely qualified to share what you know. If you don't know where to begin, buy or borrow from the library books that show step-by-step how to capture the data and stories of ancestors and your own contemporary family members. Even if you have only limited information and memories, you can still gather information on your ancestors' countries of origin, especially during the time they lived there, and learn with your grandchildren about that country's culture and history.

You can also have fun describing some of your own experiences and antics as a child. Resist the temptation to lecture your grandchildren that

"In my day, we had no TV, and I had to walk 10 miles to school in the snow, uphill both ways and barefoot." Instead, tell them about a time you were punished for misbehaving, about some award you may have won or a story about when you got lost the first time your parents had you go to the store for a loaf of bread (that cost only a penny or two, of course!).

Grandkids of all ages love to hear about their grandparents' antics and adventures. They also love to hear stories about their own parents—especially stories their parents may find too embarrassing to reveal! (Although you may want to exercise at least some discretion here, lest you make your adult children angry.)

Grandparents also may want to ensure that they impart their values to the younger generation in this changing and uncertain world. Often, when both parents work, they may not have enough time to give their children the guidance they need.

In response to the AARP 2002 grandparent survey's open-ended question about the most important values or ethics grandparents would like to pass on to their grandchildren, 42% said high morals and integrity, 21% cited success or ambition, 20% mentioned religion, 14% pointed to consideration of others and 10% said to be responsible or trustworthy.

Redefining Your Self-Image and Your Role as a Grandparent

Those round-number milestones—reaching your 40th, 50th, 60th birthdays, etc.—can be tough to pass gracefully. But when that first grandchild comes into the picture, many people, especially those who have always identified themselves as part of the youth or boomer generation, can no longer deny that their youth is, well, gone. Perhaps not their youthfulness, but certainly their youth.

Still, becoming an older person in today's world, as I've already mentioned, is quite different than when our own grandparents hit the grandparent milestone. If you carry a cane, it's likely stylish—a fashion statement as well as a functional necessity. While some spirited oldsters—the late actress Ruth Gordon comes to mind—bucked the old-fart, out-of-touch-with-contemporary-culture stereotypical granny, many people smile condescendingly at her energy and antics, thinking, "Isn't she adorable?"

Pu-leeze! Today we are not adorable, we're simply vibrant. We're as capable as anyone half our age of doing just about anything. If there was one consoling image post-September 11th, for me it was hearing stories of airport security personnel signaling people young and old, of both genders, off the check-point line to be more thoroughly searched. Yes, we old geezers can even be dangerous!

In terms of our roles as grandparents, I feel no societal constraints to fit any traditional and passé grandpersona. In fact, becoming a grandparent has thoroughly liberated me to be as playful—perhaps even immature—as I want to be, and I feel proud of it! Tempered with all the wisdom we hope we have acquired over the years, aging and grandparenthood can make these years exciting and fulfilling.

However, we're usually not in this role alone. Grandparents are part of a system. Picture three concentric circles, at the center of which are the grandchildren, then their parents and then the grandparents. We are used to calling the shots in our family, but we're no longer in charge. So, one of the first ways to get grandparenting off to a good start is to stake out the boundaries. Don't step on your adult children's toes; respect their authority and the decisions they make concerning childrearing. And never undermine those decisions, no matter how wrong you think they are!

On the other hand, you are also perfectly free to buck many entrenched beliefs, expectations and demands your adult children may try to impose on you about your role as grandparents. When I interviewed Susan Kettmann on my radio show, she described some of the expectations she addressed in her book, *The 12 Rules of Grandparenting: A New Look at Traditional Roles and How to Break Them* (Facts on File, 2000). For instance, Kettmann takes issue with the notion that grandparents love to babysit.

You may have an active life, and as much as you may love to visit your grandchildren, you may not want or feel up to providing regular childcare and all that goes with it—diapers, drool and blood-curdling screams. "Look at all those expectations," urges Kettmann, "and don't be afraid to say, 'This is expecting a lot of one person.' For some people, babysitting is what they've been waiting for. Others are nervous, have medical conditions, may have a full life and not want to give up all their free time. Don't worry, 'What will they think if I don't babysit?' There are lots of other ways to show grandchildren and your children that you love them."

If you do feel able and willing to babysit, consider negotiating a written agreement to make sure both you and your adult children are clear about what you will and won't do and when you will or won't do it.

Other issues you may want to spell out are what circumstances under which you will call the parents at work. Do your adult children want you to call immediately if the baby takes her first step? (If so, resist gloating that you were the first to witness that step!) Do the parents want to wait until they get home to learn about an ugly diaper rash or a low-grade fever? If so, make sure you have the name and number of the pediatrician, and that you know how to get to the doctor's office!

Kettmann also suggests that if you are babysitting in your own home, that you create a place where the children know there are things they can play with. Don't be afraid to give even little toddlers some chores: children love to help out, and if they are busy dusting or washing a dish or two, you can keep your eyes on them while you're preparing lunch or making some needed phone calls. Kettman provides a list of suggested chores in her book. She points out another benefit: "Even letting them help you make cookies or work in the garden is something they'll remember all their lives." Dr. Ruth emphasizes that some grandparents may be able to help pay for tuition or vacations, while others are having too hard a time with their own financial struggles. "But we all have one thing in common—we love our grandchildren and want to help them. It has nothing to do with income or race."

She also points out some possible land mines in the grandparent territory, such as how to celebrate holidays when the parents have two different religions, or how to deal with divorce, remarriage and step grandchildren. Be up-front and direct with your adult children and their spouse about how to navigate these issues. And never forget—even though the next section deals with spoiling the grandchildren—that you can never spoil them with too much love!

Spoiling Grandkids

Grandparents spend about $30 billion a year on their grandchildren. Some stores say grandparents now account for more than a third of all its kiddie-gear sales. That's a 20% jump in the last five years. The latest trend is buying for grandchildren online. Analysts estimate that by 2005, grandparents will purchase $15 billion worth of goods and services over the Internet.

So it shouldn't come as much surprise that the most common complaint that adult children hurl at their parents is, "They're undermining everything I'm trying to accomplish. I try to teach them some discipline and my parents spoil my kids rotten!" On the other hand, the most common complaint grandparents have about the way their adult kids are raising their grandchildren goes something like this: "They're doing a horrible job, sending all the wrong signals about money. They're spoiling my grandchildren rotten!"

Jayne Pearl, author of *Kids and Money: How to Give Them the Savvy to Succeed Financially* (Bloomberg Press, 1999), says she would dole out the same advice to both generations: "Get over it. Don't worry. Relax. There's not much you can do to control what the other one does; but your own actions and behavior can still exert a very positive influence on the kids."

For the parents with indulgent grandparents, Pearl says, "Don't be such a party pooper! Trying to put a damper on lavish gifts will only make you the bad guy. The grandparents resent you for impinging on their pleasure in giving. You won't earn any brownie points from your kids. However, if you remain clear and consistent about your own financial parenting rules, your lessons will not be diminished by what they receive from others. Remind your kids that even though you don't approve of everything their grandparents give them, it gives both giver and receiver pleasure, and you're confident your kids can understand that doesn't change the rules under your roof."

For grandparents whose grown children are doing it all wrong, Pearl advises to give it up. "Even if you're completely correct," she points out, "your days of influencing what your own children do are over (if they ever existed at all!). But you can still exert a wonderful, positive influence over your grandchildren. Even if their parents indulge their every fancy, you can initiate some fun and meaningful projects with them that can leave lasting impressions."

For instance, Pearl suggests you introduce them to the world of investing. Buy them one or more shares in some public company (preferably, one that is tied to one of your grandchildren's interests—such as in McDonald's or Disney) or mutual fund or join or start an investment club together. You can spend visits, phone calls or e-mails with your grandkids tracking the investment's performance, exploring new investments and discussing what you are each learning.

We cannot control what others do. Instead of wasting our energy and breath trying to force change, come up with creative ways to temper even the most egregious parenting or grandparenting faux pas.

Raising Your Grandchildren

Grandparents' visitation rights have become a focal point of attention with the Supreme Court's Troxel v. Granville decision in June 2000 to deny a grandparent's petition for visitation rights with their grandchildren.

However, an equally disturbing trend can be found at the other end of the spectrum: when grandparents end up having to assume primary care for their grandchildren.

The recent Census found that 4.5 million children live in grandparent-headed households. About one-third of these children have no parents living with them. Researchers report that at some point, one in 10 grandparents will find themselves raising one or more grandchildren for at least six months. However, grandparents can take on that responsibility for far longer periods, possibly five years or more.

Grandmothers are typically the caregivers, but in 6% of the grandparent-headed households, grandfathers were the sole caregiver.

Grandparents often step in after a grandchild's parent loses contact with the child or ends up in jail, but the top reasons are substance abuse, teenage pregnancy, divorce and mental illness. Other grandparents assume responsibility when a child's parents die.

Most grandparents had not planned to spend their golden years returning to the parent role. What a shock to go from the delightful role of being able to dote on your grandchildren to having to assume the responsibility of disciplining and raising them!

One major challenge is money. Many care-giving grandparents live on fixed incomes, and have an annual income of $18,000—half that of a traditional two-parent home.

But help is available. For instance, many states provide some form of Temporary Assistance to Needy Families. Your state's Social Security Office or Area Agency on Aging—both should be listed in the blue pages of your phone book—can tell you whether such a program, or other forms of financial assistance, exist in your area. The National Family Caregiver Support Program (http://www.aoa.gov/caregivers), a federally funded effort to help family members provide care for the elderly at home, offers services for caregivers who are 60 or older.

Caregiving grandparents who are not legal custodians or guardians of their grandchildren may find it hard to secure the basic services their grandchildren need. However, becoming a legal custodian or guardian is a time-consuming, expensive and emotionally exhausting process. It's wise to hire an attorney. Adopting one's grandchildren is the most difficult approach, requiring that the parent(s) relinquish their legal parental rights or that the court declares the parent(s) legally incompetent. During an adoption process, the child becomes a temporary ward of the state.

The most common questions new care-giving grandparents pose include:

• What are my legal and financial rights?

• What rights do grandparents have if they are not legal guardians?

• Can adult children just show up some day and take my grandchildren back?

Each state has its own laws that address these questions. For information on visitation, custody and adoption and how to find out the laws in your state, contact Grandparents United for Children's Rights, Inc. (608-238-5115; 137 Larkin Street, Madison, WI 53705).

Grandparents who suddenly find themselves returning to childcare may experience a wide range of emotions, such as feelings of guilt, helplessness and isolation. Grandparents also have to deal with their grandchildren's anxieties about being separated from their biological parents.

Another area of concern: Grandparents' physical health can erode as a result of the stress from caring for young children. They often neglect their own physical and emotional health when they devote their attention and energy on their grandchildren's needs. But this is short-sighted. As tough as it may be to attend to both sets of needs, consider the consequences of the grandparents becoming incapacitated and unable to nurture their grandchildren.

Support groups can help, by providing information and friendship. Such groups are most successful when they provide activities for the grandchildren to do while their grandparents meet. Your local Area Agency on Aging can help you locate any grandparenting support groups in your region. For grandparents living in areas that don't have such groups, Internet chat rooms can connect grandparents 24 hours a day to other grandparents raising grandchildren.

Other Resources:

Books

The Essential Grandparent, by Dr. Lillian Carson (Health Communications, 1997)

To Grandmother's House We... Stay, by Sally Houtman (Studio 4 Productions Publishing, 1999)

Grownups' Guide to Computing, by Mary Furlong, Stephan Lipson and Craig Spiezle (Microsoft Press, 1999)

The 12 Rules of Grandparenting: A New Look at Traditional Roles and How to Break Them, by Susan M. Kettmann (Facts on File publisher, 2000).

Organizations

AARP Grandparent Information Center
www.aarp.org/grandparents
A portal chock full of articles, information and suggestions concerning fun,

gift-giving, computers, health and safety, grandparent visitation, and resources for grandparents raising grandchildren.

Generations Unlimited
www.gu.org
Focuses solely on promoting intergenerational strategies, programs and policies via 100 national, state and local organizations representing more than 70 million Americans.

Grand Parent Again
www.grandparentagain.com
Provides information and support concerning legal and medical issues and an online forum with discussion groups for grandparents who are parenting their grandchildren.

GrandsPlace
www.grandsplace.com
Another site for grandparents parenting grandkids. This one promises a safe and accepting environment where caregivers can join together and give each other the support and comfort they need.

National Council on Aging
www.ncoa.org
The nation's first association of organizations and professionals dedicated to promoting the dignity, self-determination, well being and contributions of older persons. NCOA is a private, nonprofit group that advocates for public policies, societal attitudes and business practices that promote vital aging; conducts research geared to creation of effective programs and services to serve seniors.

Chapter 8

How to Afford or Avoid Retirement

Before World War II, retirement was all but unheard of. You literally worked until you dropped. In fact, as Peter G. Peterson points out in *Gray Dawn* (Crown Publishers, 1999), the word "retirement" used to have a negative connotation. It implied that one's useful days were over. Men stayed on the job whether they could afford to retire or not.

Then, after the Depression, President Roosevelt initiated the Social Security Act to provide a safety net—to protect retirees from poverty. Over time, Social Security expanded to provide benefits to all retirees, regardless of income or wealth.

During World War II, when there were more jobs than workers, employers used fringe benefits, such as pensions, to attract and keep workers without violating the wartime wage-freeze rules. The rise of pension plans and health benefits for former employees swiftly made retirement an appealing option. Retirement has become a socially accepted, even celebrated phase of life.

In fact, since the fifties, workers have been retiring at ever-younger ages. In the early 1950s, the average age of retirement for men was 68.5 years; for women 67.9.[1] Those rates steadily declined, reaching 62.9 for both men and women in the early 1970s, then leveled off for the next two decades and began slightly declining again during the 1990s, to 62.6.

Lower retirement ages, coupled with longer life spans, means Americans are spending more years of their lives in retirement: from 12 years (men) and 13.6 years (women) in the early 1990s to 18 years (men) and 21.7 years (women) in the period 1995 to 2000.

Women often have more reason to save, plan and, perhaps, worry. Women typically earn on average 20% to 30% less than men, and their work years are often interrupted while they raise children or care for aging parents. The result is they pay less into Social Security and private pension plans, which will diminish their sources of future retirement income by an average of $659,130. Divorce can also cause women to experience decreased income and assets, especially if they are not aware of all marital assets to which they're entitled.

Early Retirement: A Fading Dream?

Baby boomers are going to rewrite the way we view retirement. At the very least, baby boomers might be working more years than their parents did. Some because they have to, some because they want to.

Some take on second or third careers. Mickey Rooney, for instance, well into his eighties, told listeners of *A Touch of Grey*, "I say don't retire, inspire." He is still on the road performing, but also writes. In addition to his memoir, *Life is Too Short* (Villard Books, 1991), Rooney penned a mystery novel, *Search for Sonny Skies* (Birch Lane Press, 1994).

Another guest on *A Touch of Grey*, Jack LaLanne, is also active well into his eighties. "The minute your physical condition is good, your mind works better," he told listeners.

Many folks find meaning in their jobs, and have even wrapped their identity in their work. They wouldn't dream of retiring. They wouldn't know what to do and would have a difficult time adjusting to open-ended days, without having to get dressed and combat rush hour to get to the office. They intend to work as long as possible.

I plan to be one of them. I never want to retire completely—I'll work part-time, talking and consulting about senior issues. Five or 10 years from now I may not necessarily have my own radio show, but I can envision going on and being an expert on other people's shows, talking about whatever issues concern older Americans at that particular time. I also want to encourage other women in their careers.

Being a guest on other radio and television talk shows will allow me to work a more flexible schedule. Currently, I get up at 4:30 am, look at the newspapers, find out the latest news concerning the guests scheduled to appear on my show that day. I'll read their books and make sure I'm prepared before I go on the air. That takes a lot of time and effort. I enjoy doing it now, but I can see myself winding down eventually.

The movie, *About Schmidt*, opens with Jack Nicholson's character attending his own, somewhat surreal retirement party. He seems outwardly numb and awkward, inwardly terrified and disgusted through the event, dreading the empty days that he knows will follow. In real life, Nicholson, who was 65 when the movie came out in 2003, admits his own mixed feelings about retiring. He told *Newsweek*, "I have had a charmed life. I got to do most of what I ever wanted to do. I mean, I started thinking about quitting acting a little while ago. You think, 'Who wants to see anything I would do? Who cares?' It was regular depressive thinking, where you're down on yourself and you think you're not growing. But then I remembered why I started acting: I'm not happy if I'm not expressive."[2] Even though most of us don't get to live lives as charmed as his or enjoy careers as glamorous as his we also might dread confronting the void that retirement seems to represent for so many of us.

Retirement is bound to change the rhythms of our lives. Although retirement may provide time to relax and pursue interests we could not do while we were working and raising a family, the sudden lack of a schedule and built-in social life can wreak havoc on our emotions and also on our relationships. As one wife said of her husband after he retired, "I married him for better or for worse, but not for lunch."

The decision whether to retire or keep working is a personal one. There's no right or wrong today. Today's increasingly healthy and vital retirees may prefer rock climbing to rocking chairs. Only you know the combination of family, health, financial and other variables that will determine what's best for you. The great thing about retirement is that you can change your mind any time. If your finances or feelings reverse at any time, you can always resume or halt working. Or, like I plan to do, you can have the best of both worlds and semi-retire—continue working part-time, and have increased time to relax, travel, volunteer, visit the grandkids, take courses or master new technology.

What happens if you think you'd like to retire, but you're not sure if you can afford to? Economic turmoil may make it harder not just to retire early, but at all! You may have any or all of these three main forces to thank: increased demands on your financial resources; lack of sufficient planning and saving, and erosion of the value of what you have saved. Let's take a closer look at these economic and social forces.

Increased Demands on Our Financial Resources

For instance, as we age, it's reasonable to expect our health-care needs to increase. At the same time, health insurance costs are rising dramatically, and policies are covering less, even as medical costs are also increasing for prescriptions, tests, hospital stays and doctors' visits. And as we will discuss in Chapter 11, Medicare coverage is also diminishing. One positive ray: While we will have to spend more on health care during our retirement years, our living expenses will likely drop more than medical bills will rise. Ironically, working longer may have a positive impact on our health as well as our wallets, both in terms of more income and lower health-care expenses. That's because some experts claim that a longer work life will improve the health of older Americans. Leading American Gerontologist Dr. Robert Butler has said we must develop a vision of "productive aging" in which "work expectancy" rises along with "life expectancy." He went on to say if people desire satisfying sex at age 70, why not satisfying work as well?

Many baby boomers are also members of the "sandwich generation," meaning that they are enduring maximum financial stress. Many are concurrently paying for their children's education, planning for retirement, and supporting elderly parents. Many experts recommend that you save for retirement first, and then worry about college. "You can borrow for college (or your kids can), but you can't live on loans in your old age," says personal financial columnist Jane Bryant Quinn.[3] If you do retire while your kids are in college, your income will drop, which will make them eligible for more tuition aid.

Living longer than any other previous generation also means we must have the financial resources to meet our own extended needs. However, Social Security and Medicare were not designed to match the boomer generation's size and extended longevity. According to a recent Age Wave/Roper poll, 90% of boomers believe that the government has made financial promises that it will be unable to keep. They are not just cynical; they have every reason to feel concerned—but not for 30 years, at least. If no changes are made to the program, come the 2030s, retirees will receive less than 75% of their benefits (in tomorrow's inflation-adjusted dollars). However, since its introduction in 1935, Social Security has been reliable, paying every benefit check, on time, every month, every year.

Social Security: Who, When, How Much?

To qualify for Social Security, individuals or couples must be U.S. citizens (with some exceptions), age 65 or older, blind or disabled. The amount of the benefit depends on the income the individual or couple receives.

To find out how much you can expect to receive, get a copy of your Social Security statement, which estimates the size of your benefit if you start at age 62, normal retirement age (probably 65 or 66) or 70. If you don't have a current statement, you can order one by phone at 800-772-1213 or online at www.ssa.gov to order one.

In the early 1900s, life expectancy was 47.3 years. Today, it has reached a record high of 76.9 years. In 1950, there were 16 productive workers to each retiree. That number has shrunk today to just 3.3. These numbers simply mean that a decreasing number of workers won't be able to adequately support baby boomers as they reach old age.

Unfortunately, many people today don't realize that Social Security, even with its extended coverage, was never intended to be the sole means of support for retired workers. The government always assumed that individuals would supplement their Social Security income with other built-up financial assets. But Americans are woefully lax on this front.

Lack of Sufficient Planning and Saving

We are also lax when it comes to our awareness of keeping track of money we may have from a previous job's pension plan. It may pay off handsomely to contact previous employers to learn the status of your benefits and how you can receive them. Or you can contact the Pension Benefits Guaranty Corp. (www.pbgc.gov or 202-326-4000), a government-chartered agency that can help you search for such benefits.

Today's workers are clearly overly optimistic and out of sync with reality. In a recent study by The American Savings Education Council, 70% of workers 40 to 59 said they were confident they would be able to have a comfortable retirement. Yet only 25% had saved at least $100,000. Half of all workers have saved less than $50,000 and 15% report that they have saved nothing.

One third of baby boomers are well off. They are earning large salaries, have invested profitably, and will be lucky enough to be the major part of the population that receives a $10 trillion inheritance from the preceding generation.

Another third will have to extend their work life at least five years beyond their current expectations, to have a satisfactory retirement.

The last third, largely female, have virtually no savings, no investments, no pensions, and are unlikely to receive any inheritance.

Of course, the best prescription for retiring well is to have a disciplined saving plan in place. Unfortunately, America has the lowest saving rate of any developed country in the world. Part of the problem for boomers is that they are not long-range planners. My motto, as I go through life is: it's never too late, so if you haven't got a savings plan, start one now.

Eroding Value of What We Have Saved

Unfortunately, many boomers have recently received an unpleasant financial wake-up call. The stock market's recent doldrums have resulted in many 401(k) plans, IRAs and other investments losing half their value. This fact, in connection with companies scaling back many retiree health benefits, may make many retirees reevaluate the costs of early retirement. Another major factor contributing to the precariousness of retirement comfort is ignorance. Many of the financial forces are beyond our control. However, one important factor—financial literacy—is well within our reach, yet not pursued by many. A recent study by Professor Neil Cutler of The National Council on the Aging (NCOA) found that half of boomers didn't know that Medicare doesn't pay for long-term care. Although two-thirds of boomers say they're worried about having enough money in the future, 64% say they have no idea how much money they'll need during retirement. Most experts estimate that you'll need 60% to 80% of what you now earn—per year, for 20 or more years!

Financial columnist Jane Bryant Quinn suggests this quick quiz to see if you can afford to retire: Take 5% or 6% of your total retirement savings and add other expected income, say from a part-time job. "If you can live on that for a year, you can probably wave goodbye to the job you're doing now," Quinn writes in *Newsweek*.[4]

However, if stock prices bomb for a few years right after you retire, you may need to rethink this equation. Your investments would not outlive you. You can more thoroughly estimate how big a nest egg you'll need before you can retire at Bank Rate's online retirement calculator (http://www.bankrate.com/usn/cgi-bin/Retire.asp). Here's what the calculator predicts for a 48-year-old woman earning $50,000 a year today, who wants to retire by age 67. Actuarially, the calculator estimates she can expect to live to age 95—which means she will need to support herself for 28 years after she retires.

The calculator says this woman will need $800,000 in savings to cover her retirement (assuming annual income of $38,500—77% of current income—at retirement, 2% inflation and 7.5% yield on the balance).

Obviously, saving more might not solve all her retirement problems. She, and many of us, will have to work longer. Fortunately, the Senior Citizen's Freedom to Work Act of 2000 pushes the retirement-earnings limit for Social Security beneficiaries from age 65 to 70. This makes it possible for older people to keep working without sacrificing their benefits. Although we can now choose to work and still collect, the age at which one can collect Social Security is gradually increasing, making it all the more financially necessary for many to keep working.

However, don't buy into all those reports that say you need a $1 million nest egg to retire comfortably. Georgia State University's Center for Risk Management & Insurance Research points out that a 65-year-old couple earning $50,000 a year will need pretax income of $37,000 a year to maintain their standard of living in retirement, thanks to lower costs for such things as transportation and clothing, taxes, and other expenses. Because Social Security should provide nearly $24,000 of that for the typical 65-year-old couple, they only need about $13,000 a year from savings and other sources. Even if neither partner continues to work full- or part-time, if they both live to 85, they'll need savings of less than $260,000 to meet that need.

Aging expert Ken Dychtwald, AIG SunAmerica and Harris Interactive surveyed 1,000 pre-retirees and retirees about their attitudes, which the surveyors grouped into four categories: ageless explorers (27%), comfortably contents (19%), live for todays (22%), and the sick and tireds (32%). One of the survey's strongest findings was that those who had prepared for retirement, regardless of their wealth or income, tended to be the most satisfied.

Because a little planning will go a long way, here are some ways to get started.

Getting Your Financial House in Order

• Calculate how much you will need to retire comfortably. If you're still concerned about outliving your nest egg, use the Bank Rate calculator mentioned above, or another retirement income calculator.

• Educate yourself about your financial resources—pension, 401(k)s, etc. Given the complex financial options surrounding retirement, it is probably a good idea to consult with a certified financial planner.

• Retire your credit-card debt before you retire yourself. Pay down your high-interest debt (loans and credit cards) as soon as possible. People 65 and older tripled the amount of household debt they hold since 1992, to an average $23,000, according to SRI Consulting Business Intelligence. Nearly half of seniors carry credit card balances instead of paying off their outstanding balance each month. That may contribute to why seniors are the fastest-growing group of personal bankruptcy filers.

• Start saving at least 10% of your income monthly. The stock market is unlikely to have double-digit returns again in the foreseeable future, so don't expect tremendous gains to cover all your needs. But saving will certainly help!

• Maximize all allowable tax-protected savings, such as 401(k)s to take advantage of compounding growth. Find out about the new catch-up provisions for workers 50 and older.

• Consider a reverse home mortgage (RHM). If you are home rich but cash poor, and are 62 or older and own your home free and clear or have a very small mortgage balance, you have the option of using your house as a source of tax-free income.

Unlike a traditional mortgage where you pay out a monthly sum of money, an RHM instead pays you, in the form of a lump sum or monthly payments. You can also obtain a line of credit to use when needed along with one of the payoff options. As for the interest rates, RHMs are usually offered at variable rates.

The amount of money you can receive from a reverse home mortgage depends on several factors: your age, your home's value and location and current interest rates.

The National Reverse Mortgage Lenders Association emphasizes that you are still responsible for your home's taxes, repairs and maintenance costs.

However, there are many advantages. For instance, because payments are considered a loan, they are tax-free. You can use the money for any purpose, including home improvements, in-home health care, taxes and insurance premiums. Some people, whose CDs or IRAs have been hammered by the drop in interest rates and stock prices, are opting for reverse mortgage lines of credit as a security cushion. An RHM guarantees you a source of money for as long as you need it, no matter how long you live, and you only have to pay it off when you sell the home, move out permanently or, upon your death. Once the house is sold, any surplus after the debt to the lender is paid will go to your heirs.

However, an RHM is no free lunch. They can be extremely expensive transactions, with high closing costs, monthly compounding of interest, servicing fees and mortgage insurance that rises with the loan balance. You can finance these fees, but then those costs will then be tacked on to your loan. This type of loan can also reduce the size of the estate your heirs will receive.

Low-income borrowers need to be especially careful. An RHM might make it difficult to qualify for other badly needed aid such as Supplemental Security Income or Medicaid. One other caveat: RHMs are so complex that you are required to receive counseling before applying for one.

So although RHMs can be a great alternative for some older Americans with cash-flow problems, they are not for everyone.

A recent Retirement Confidence Survey found that 51% of retirees say retirement is better than they expected; 26% say it is about the same; while 19% report it is worse than expected.

Whether you hope to retire early, at the traditional age of 65, or never, careful planning—of your finances, living situation and emotional needs—will help make sure your older years are comfortable and happy.

Other Resources:

• American Savings Education Council website
www.asec.org
Features "Savings Tools" with a variety of worksheets to help with retirement planning and saving.

• Certified Financial Planner Board of Standards' Financial Planning Resource Kit
888- 237-6275

• Cooperative Extension System, an affiliate of the U.S. Department of Agriculture
www.money2000.org.
Monitor spending and increase savings, or use their guidelines and interactive calculator to create a budget.

• Department of Housing and Urban Development's Housing Counseling Clearinghouse
888-466-3487

• National Center for Home Equity Conversion
www.reverse.org
612-953-4474

• National Council on Aging Benefits Checkup
www.benefitscheckup.org
Helps people age 55 and older find programs to help them pay for pre-

scription drugs, health care, utilities and other essential items or services.

• "Savings Fitness: A Guide to Your Money and Your Financial Future" by the U.S. Department of Labor and the Certified Financial Planner Board of Standards is available at no cost by calling 800-998-7542.

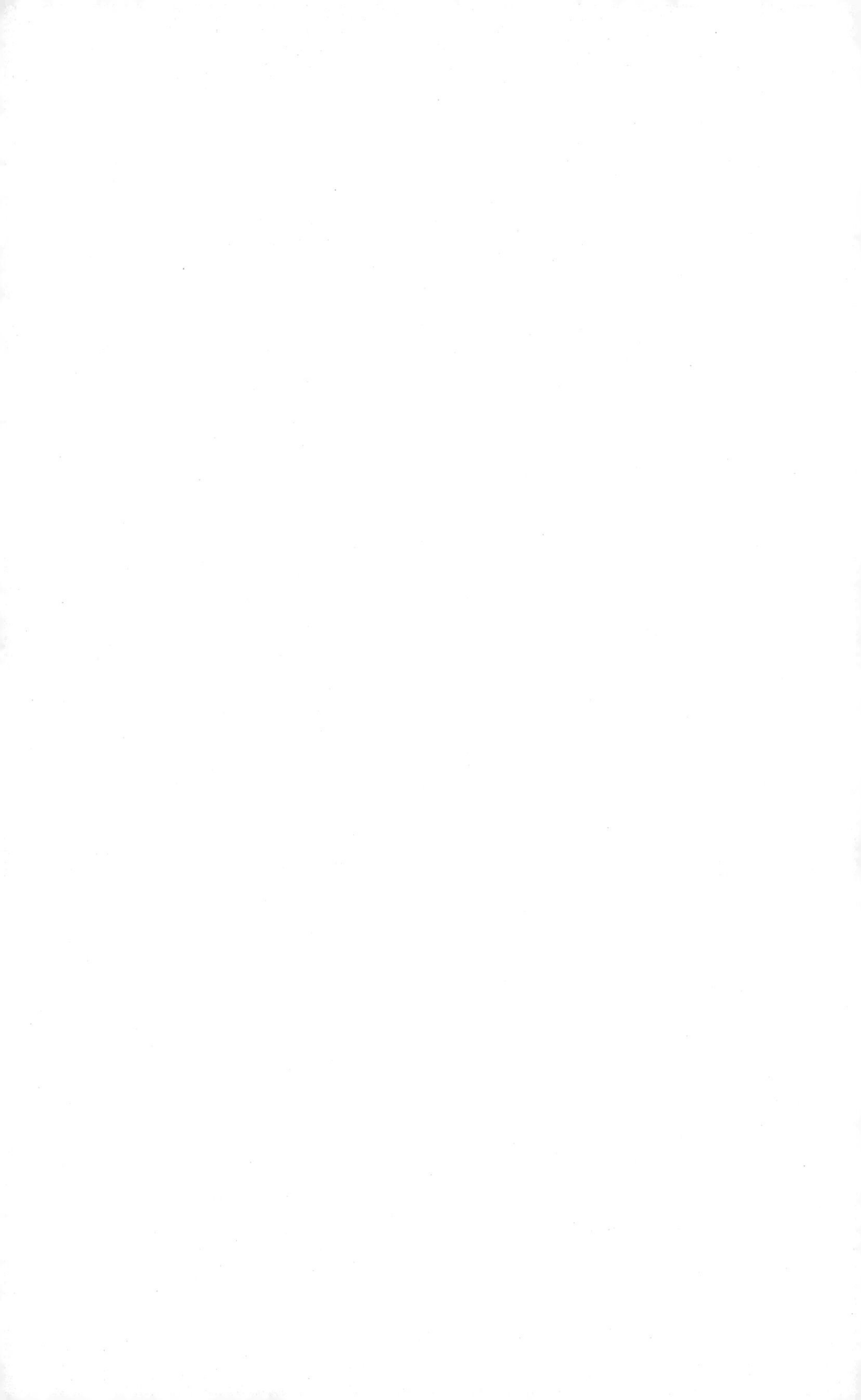

Chapter 9

*What a Long, Strange Trip It's Been:
Traveling in Style*

My Life's Odyssey

If I could point to one thing that has helped me grow as a human being and shaped my philosophy about life, it's travel. My interest in other places and cultures started with the wonderful travel books my parents gave me during my early years. In particular, one book, *The Royal Road to Romance*, by Richard Haliburton (Traveler's Tales Guides 2000), mesmerized me with its descriptions of strange and exotic countries, as I pictured myself visiting them. I was enthralled to read how Haliburton traveled so differently than most tourists.

My parents loved to travel. They often left me with my grandparents during summer vacations, so they could take extended trips. But then when I reached my teens, they started taking me with them.

These weren't just ordinary trips. I remember going through the Panama Canal on a freighter whose mission was to deliver its cargo. We often didn't get to destinations until late at night, so sightseeing was limited. One of the most unusual ocean voyages I took with my parents was on the maiden voyage of the S.S. United States. Inaugurated on July 3, 1952, she was the fastest and most modern ship of her day. En route to Europe, the ocean-liner established a new transatlantic speed record—just three days. We had to wait an extra day off the coast of France so we could disembark at the proper time and place in England.

Another memorable way we traveled long ago was on a Pan American-Grace Airways DC 6, which took us in 1951 across South America's Andes Mountains. The ride is etched in my memories for two reasons: the roughness of the trip and the use of oxygen masks as we flew over the mountains. In those days, planes did not have pressurized cabins.

Making Travel Affordable

As I grew older, my love of travel endured, although its form has changed. After I married and had four children, trips were dictated both by budget and time constraints. My adventure gene did surface, though, when I proposed that my family take a six-week drive across a good part of the country in a rented station wagon. At the time, my children spanned from teenagers to elementary schoolers. Today we all look back at our trip with a great deal of fondness.

After my divorce, with mostly grown children, I had even more limited financial resources and worked hard to support myself. I had to find more creative and less expensive ways to indulge my travel passion. Fortunately, in 1984 I landed a job in Connecticut that I found challenging and truly enjoyable. I was executive director of the Retired Senior Volunteer Program (RSVP) of Southern New London County. I recruited, trained, and placed 700 volunteers, 65 and older, in 97 non-profit agencies. Many of these women were widows who often talked about how lonely they were and how much they missed the trips they had taken with their spouses.

I came up with the idea of putting together some trips with a local travel agency and offering them to my volunteers. The trips were very popular because the volunteers would pick them, they knew each other and they felt comfortable having me as the group's leader. I took RSVP members to destinations such as Ireland, islands in the Caribbean, Hawaii, the Panama Canal and Alaska. Some of the trips were by bus, some were via a cruise boat.

It wasn't all fun, though. Being a tour guide is a huge responsibility. I once had to evacuate someone from a trip in Juneau, Alaska, which can only be reached by sea or air. She had to be flown to a hospital in Anchorage. Travel agents and tour guides should insist that travelers show their doctor a brochure of their trip, and even more important, get a note stating any medical problems and attesting to their ability to handle the rigors of a trip.

In addition to finding affordable ways to travel, you can also find other forms of entertainment for free—for instance, you can apply to become an usher at concerts and plays at local venues. Or offer to write a travel column for your local paper. If you earn money for the column, you can also write off your trip expenses! Likewise, consider becoming a local food, arts or music critic. You might be able to indulge in these fancies for free at some restaurants and theatres.

Smooth Sailing

Running trips for seniors helped me learn what they really appreciated, such as always finding someone to help them put their carry-on luggage up in the overhead bin. If you're older, this can be a very difficult task. I also did their immigration paperwork and made sure they got through airports and customs with the least hassle.

I always checked out the suitability of a trip before I offered it. Once Alitalia airlines offered me a free three-day trip to the Amalfi coast of Italy as an inducement to take a tour there and use their airline. That trip ranks as the longest distance I've ever schlepped for the shortest period of time! Here are some other tips to keep your travels trouble free:

• **Avoid E-tickets if possible.** These are computerized airline tickets that allow you to avoid check-in counter lines and proceed right to your gate to arrange your seat and collect your boarding pass. Sounds good, but if your flight is canceled, you may have a tough time exchanging an E-ticket for another airline's ticket, because E-tickets do not list your fare code. Stick with paper tickets if possible, and live with the lines.

• **But avoid the ticket-counter line to rebook a canceled flight.** Instead, use a public or your cell phone to call your airline's toll-free number to reach a phone agent who can book you on the next flight much faster.

• **Check out carry-on luggage rules before you pack your bags.** Then measure your carry-ons after you pack them, to make sure they meet your carrier's limit.

After I started *A Touch of Grey*, my syndicated radio show for those 50-plus, satellites and cell phones have enabled me to broadcast from the far reaches of mother earth and convey to my listeners the immediacy and wonder of the sights I'm seeing.

Post 9-11 Rules of the Road (and Air)

The horrific events of September 11, 2001 dealt a harsh blow to the travel industry. Yet there was a waiting list for my trip in 2003 around the world! Indeed, a lot of international travel has been picking up. For now, you may want to consider a few extra precautions to minimize risks:

• **Allow extra time.** Get to the airport or train station early. Call the airport to find out how much time before your plane's scheduled departure you should arrive. Once you get there, expect and accept that lines will be longer and nerves will be shorter. Try to go with the flow, by bringing some light, fun reading to pass the time. Also pack snacks to enjoy.

• **Insure your trip.** Many domestic and international travelers are wisely opting to buy travel insurance, to make sure you can recoup your fares, lodging, car rental and other travel costs in the event that you become ill or political events prevent you from taking your trip. Premiums can run 5% to 10% of the cost of your trip, but that's better than losing all your upfront outlays if you are forced to cancel your plans.

• **Don't overstuff your carry-on or checked bags.** You want to make it easy for security screeners to reseal your luggage if they hand inspect it, recommends the Transportation Security Administration (www.tsatraveltips.us). Wait to wrap gifts until you reach your destination, as you may have open them for screeners. Also check with your travel agent or the air line about prohibited items that could result in your being criminally and/or civilly prosecuted, or at least asked to rid yourself of them.

• **Avoid wearing metal items** such as jewelry, belts, hair clips, metal buttons, shoes with metal tips, or even under-wire bras, which may set off the alarm as you pass through the security check point. Also avoid placing change, keys or other metal items in your pocket. Place such items in your carry-on bag until you go through security.

Beating Jet Lag and Other Health Hazards

As security checks at airports and most tourist spots have escalated dramatically, the resulting increases in travel time can be especially grueling for seniors. It's more important today than ever to make sure that you are not only safe from terrorists, but also from jet lag and potential health hazards that air and ground travel can pose. What do you need to do in flight (or on board a bus or train or in the car) to make sure you feel as good when you get to your destination as you did when you got on?

• **Demand fresh air.** Many passengers disembark the plane with a stuffy nose, headache or the beginning of some airborne contagious illness. One of the main culprits is the lack of regulations governing the ratio of outside fresh air and re-circulated air in the cabin. Airlines are therefore free to promote fuel efficiency and reduce costs by reducing the amount of fresh air that is piped into the passenger cabin—unless passengers speak out and complain, suggests retired flight attendant Diana Fairchild in her book *Jet Smart* (Celestial Arts, 1994). You can keep other people's germs at bay by asking the flight attendant to request that the pilot allow "full utilization of air," an airline term that will let the pilot know you are an informed consumer.

• **Avoid drinking any alcohol.** The impact of alcohol on the body is two to three times more potent when you're flying. One glass of wine in-flight has the effect of two to three glasses on the ground.

• **Drink plenty of water.** The dry air in the cabin does cause dehydration.

• **Eat lightly.** Seating in a cramped position puts extra pressure on your stomach, so it's wise not to keep it full. As for that airline coffee—not only does it tend to taste awful but it often has a higher than usual caffeine content.

• **S-t-r-e-t-c-h.** If I'm on a flight of more than two hours I always do some stretching exercises in my seat, to ward off potential blood clots.

- **Clean your own space.** In her book, *Flying Blind, Flying Safe* (Harper Collins, 1997), Mary Schiavo, a former inspector general of the U.S. Department of Transportation, reveals that planes are not kept terribly clean. No regulations require the airlines to launder the blankets, replace the pillows, disinfect or even wipe off the tray tables. Many flights have such short turn-arounds that they don't have time to do any housekeeping chores. What can you do? Bring your own sealed disinfectant hand wipes to wipe off the tray tables and arm rests.

Be sure to keep airline blankets away from your nose, mouth and eyes. Finally if you like to use a pillow, carry your own inflatable neck pillow.

There's a lot you can do to improve your comfort and health in flight. But if you suddenly get ill while 30,000 feet above the ground, you will benefit from tremendous improvements in airline medical services. The airline industry today uses telemedicine to diagnose sick airline patients. Doctors on the ground help flight crews decide if they have a true emergency on hand and need to divert the plane. A recent study by the *Journal of Aviation, Space and Environmental Medicine* found that the diagnosis of sick fliers by doctors was on target with the post-landing diagnoses.

The FAA recently ruled that all passenger planes must carry defibrillators, which can, in many cases, restart a heart that has stopped beating.

Taking the Grandkids

Traveling with your grandchildren can be extremely rewarding. You can bond much more closely with them as you experience an adventure and learn about new places and people together. But it can also be taxing, especially if you have not thought through all the needs, issues and emotional baggage (no pun intended!) that are bound to surface.

Many travel agencies and tour operators have spotted an opportunity in changing demographics—namely, that today's grandparents are healthier and wealthier and more numerous than previous generations. The travel industry is beginning to capitalize on that by creating travel opportunities for intergenerational travel. Organizations such as Elderhostel (www.elderhostel.org), Grandtravel (www.grandtrvl.com) and Rascals in Paradise (www.rascalsinparadise.com) offer travel packages that cater to the needs of younger and older traveling companions.

Here are some important tips if you decide to venture off somewhere with your grandchildren:

- **Plan the trip together.** Mapping out the itinerary not only guarantees that you will choose a destination and activities that truly interest your grandchildren, but planning can be a fun and bonding experience in itself. Keep in mind that kids may miss their parents and friends and feel homesick. Keeping them busy with plenty of activities will give them less time to feel sad and pout. However, build in some flexibility to your schedule, to allow for naps, bad weather and other contingencies. The younger the children, the shorter the trip should be.

- **Take just one or two grandchildren at a time.** This will make the trip easier on everyone. It will minimize sibling squabbling, and allow you to devote more attention to each grandchild.

- **Bring plenty of healthy snacks and water.** Keep their tummies satisfied with granola bars, dried fruit, cheese, crackers and nuts, and quench their thirst with water, not soda—they sip water when they're thirsty (but will drink soda or juice to satisfy a sweet tooth). And if they don't drink too much, they will need fewer pit stops along the way.

- **Take along a supply of books, coloring or notebooks, crayons, games and music** for the plane, train or car. But leave any valuables at home. You may want to try to talk them out of taking portable video games, expensive jewelry and treasured items that can easily be lost or left on a plane.

- **Keep in contact with their parents.** Have them call their parents whenever you reach a new destination to minimize worry at both ends. Different children will feel more or less homesick when they hear their mom's or dad's voice, but let them know they can call just about any time. You can even ask parents of younger children to read a favorite story onto an audiocassette, so they can hear their parents' voice whenever they feel the need. Also, make sure the parents have your itinerary and contact information, and that you have theirs.

- **Consider bringing a journal** for you to write in together, as well as a camera.

Round Trips: My Adventures Around the Globe

One of the first trips I took after I started my radio career was a very unusual train expedition on Russia's vast Trans-Siberian Railway, sponsored by an organization of train lovers. I adore trains, and my idea for this trip sprang from the 1965 movie *Doctor Zhivago*, in which one scene was shot from a train crossing the vast steppes of Russia. It showed thousands of flowers—mostly daffodils—in bloom, an incredibly romantic image. However, this trip, across the plains from Moscow to Irkutsk, Siberia, was anything but romantic. Instead of daffodils, I encountered dust. Tons of dust, which seeped into every corner of the train and covered my clothes, even my hair. After many long days of travel, I realized why invaders from Napoleon to Hitler had failed to conquer this country: The distances across Russia are so great that it becomes increasingly difficult to supply an advancing army.

When I arrived in Siberia, I was quite surprised to find how beautiful it was in the summertime. Irkutisk is located on magnificent Lake Baikal, which is the size of Switzerland. Irkutisk had the most unusual bathrooms I've ever encountered. The shower was not enclosed. When it was on, the whole bathroom got cleaned. The bathroom was so pitched that when I shut off the shower, the water instantly ran into a drain on the floor.

My Russian trip included a short but memorable trip to Magnolia. I flew there on a tiny airplane. The runway was the desert. My lodging was a round native hut called a Yurt, which was heated by a central pit that contained logs. In the cold desert night, to keep warm, I had to keep putting logs on the fire—a ritual not conducive to sleeping.

While traveling among these nomadic people, I also experienced a desert storm. It resembles the blinding whiteout of a blizzard accompanied by biting particles of sand.

In my travels, I have broadcast from a number of isolated places. One of the coldest and most remote locations was Antarctica. The trip took place in February 2000 aboard a small ship, the M.S. Explorer. It carried

110 passengers and 65 crew.

During both legs of the voyage to and from the South Pole, we cruised the infamous Drake Passage. This body of water off the tip of South America lived up to its terrifying reputation. In the ship's log book, the captain described the ship as pitching and rolling heavily with swells ranging from eight to 25 feet. I spent the better part of two days crawling around on the cabin floor.

The South Pole gives birth to much of the world's weather. Both the winds and the atmospheric conditions are constantly changing. It's therefore a natural lab for studying global warming. When I was in Antarctica, I saw dramatic evidence of this. For example, I saw a fissure opening on the huge Larsen Ice Shelf, which is gradually disintegrating.

Using Zodiacs (little rubber rafts that Jacques Cousteau made famous), I explored a number of islands around the Antarctic Peninsula. What most surprised me about icebergs was they came in a variety of beautiful colors, including a vivid blue, pink, and green. This is caused by some of the minerals that get captured in the icebergs.

I have also broadcast from areas that were remote and hot. I have very fond memories of talking on air about the beauties of an African sunset, from a boat on the Zambezi River in Zimbabwe. I have also been able to call in to *A Touch of Grey* from South Africa's legendary blue train, one of the most luxurious trains in the world.

In an effort to see Africa's animals up front and personal, in January 2001 I went on a safari to Kenya and Tanzania. I'll never forget driving in an open Land Cruiser in the middle of thousands and thousands of zebra and wildebeest amid their annual migration through the Serengeti Plains. Buzzards and vultures hovered overhead waiting to swoop down on any animals that might not make it.

The highlight of my safari in Tanzania was driving into Ngorongoro Crater, the world's largest intact, inactive volcanic crater covering 3,200 square miles within its 600-meter walls. Lions, gazelles, rhinos, wildebeest, zebras, and elephants thrive in the crater's variety of habitats, from grassland plains, swamps, lakes, rivers and forests, to arid areas with drifting dunes.

Finding animals roaming around in other parts of Africa was a matter of luck. You could go hours without a sighting. After seeing life in the wild, I am working harder than ever for several organizations that are trying to save the world's endangered species from further encroachment by the human race.

I have made several around-the-world trips by plane. One of the countries I visited that touched me was Vietnam. I spent some in time in Hanoi, its beautiful capital. Despite the massive bombing of North Vietnam from 1965 to 1968, many beautiful buildings remain along with lovely tree-lined boulevards. It was the most bustling, energetic city I have ever seen. Getting around Hanoi was an adventure. With virtually no traffic lights, no policemen and thousands and thousands of mopeds, somehow everyone seemed to safely get where they were going.

Going through Hoa Lo, also known as the "Hanoi Hilton," which had been a brutal jail for American prisoners of war (including Senator John McCain, who was held there for more than five years), was quite an experience. It has been turned into a museum about the "American War," which is what the Vietnamese call it. Although I didn't agree with their one-sided view of the war, I did come away realizing why they fought so hard against foreigners and for their independence. The list of countries that invaded and occupied Vietnam throughout the course of history is long.

The Vietnamese people were surprisingly upbeat and friendly. Perhaps it is because instead of dwelling on past injustices that have so devastated the country, its people are concentrating on building a better future.

Finally, always seeing the glass half full, I have to comment on the wonderful island in the Indian Ocean called Mauritius. Thirty miles long and 24 miles wide, it has a remarkable mixture of cultures and religions. Dutch, French, English, Indian, Creole and Orientals, Hindus, Moslems, and Christians all live peacefully side by side in an atmosphere of great religious tolerance. If only the world could emulate the conduct of these people who live on a little island in a big ocean, we would have a more peaceful and productive world for all to enjoy.

Travel makes you realize that despite unsettling differences that are sometimes emphasized by world leaders, in the long run people are really the same. They all want peace, good health and a better future for their children.

Every trip I've taken has changed my life—especially the way I look at the world. Being a very adventurous person, I usually choose tours that include both unique and historic sites. When I learned about a trip to 12 of the United Nations Educational, Scientific, and Cultural Organization's designated historic sites, I couldn't wait to sign on.

Two of the destinations on the trip were places I had wanted to see since I was eight years old. At that tender age my mother had given me that wonderful book, *Royal Road to Romance* by Richard Halliburton. His poetic description of the Taj Mahal ignited my passion to see this masterpiece of Muslim architecture, inspired by an undying love. Haliburton also described the wonder and mystery of the world's largest religious monument, Angkor Wat, in Cambodia. My desire to visit Angkor Wat was reinforced when I learned that Jacqueline Kennedy had wanted to visit it so much when her husband was president, that she made a rare solo visit there.

Did my trip live up to my expectations? First, the Taj Mahal. You only realize how huge it is when you see it. It took 22,000 workers 18 years to build, 350 years ago. I will never forget its beauty and remarkable symmetry. Fortunately, the Taj Mahal's beautiful white marble, inlaid with semi precious stones, is not porous and has been able to withstand the densely polluted atmosphere that surrounds it.

How Foreign Seniors Fare

Everywhere I travel, I try to find out what the quality of life is for older people. In the case of India, experts expect about 40% of its growing senior population will be living below the poverty line by the year 2040. In this era of unraveling nuclear families and working families, many Indian elders in the cities are feeling lonely and are experiencing neglect. Experts feel the Indian government should draw up economic and social security programs for the elderly.

In the northern rural part of India, families are generally large and live together. The elderly are both respected and cared for by their families. What most surprised me was finding the caste system alive and well. The job you hold and the person you will marry are all determined by the caste into which you are born.

In Cambodia, I saw amazingly few senior citizens in the capitol Phnom

Penh and in the countryside. One only sees young people. More than 41% of the population is 14 or younger; almost 56% are between 15 and 64 years old, and just 3.5% are 65 or older, and life expectancy today is just 57.[1] The reason, of course, is that during the Cambodian revolution, the Khmer Rouge practiced genocide. For the four years they were in power starting in 1978, city workers were turned into farmers and everyone with skills or education was eliminated. Between one million and two million Cambodians died under the Khmer Rouge.

Cambodia is now struggling to reinvent and revitalize itself. Tourism is important and many tourists like myself come to see Angkor Wat and its intricate and delicate carvings decorate the sandstone and granite rock walls. I only saw a small section of this Hindu temple complex because it stretches over 75 square miles of jungle. Amazingly, Angkor Wat has survived invasion, abandonment, oblivion, and modern warfare. Today, one can still see the bullet holes left by the Khmer Rouge.

I also traveled to a number of other developing countries, including Ethiopia, Guatemala, and Peru. When trying to look at the quality of life for Ethiopia's elders, I faced a unique challenge. How do you define old age when life expectancy in this country is 43 years for men and 45 for women? Believe it or not, in a country of 65 million, there are only 1,600 physicians. In both India and Ethiopia, leprosy and glaucoma have yet to be eradicated. Ethiopia is also experiencing a terrible drought. The United Nations is keeping many of its aid workers away from some of the stricken areas, where rebel forces are still active.

In other countries, such as Catholic Guatemala and Peru, the traditional family remains intact and elders are respected and cared for. These countries' poor economies, however, often put a great strain on family life. For example, about half of all Peruvians live in poverty.

What a stark contrast to the changing lifestyle of more fortunate seasoned citizens from industrialized nations in the 21st century! I had had to look no further than my fellow travelers on the trip—a journey that the travel brochure described as strenuous. I would call it grueling. Often, after getting up at 5:00 am, hopping on a flight of four or five hours, upon arrival we would immediately undertake an arduous sightseeing tour. Many of my fellow travelers, in their seventies or eighties, were not a bit fazed by the schedule. The oldest person, an 85-year-old woman, was traveling on her own. She was an inspiration. The tour leaders offered walking groups designated according to ability. I never saw this seasoned citizen in the slower walking group!!

Unexpected Delights

Sometimes on a trip, you come to a place that is an unexpected surprise and delight. On this trip it was Malta. Sitting on a strategic spot in the Mediterranean, Malta has been invaded by a slew of countries, sometimes in the name of religion. The Phoenicians, Romans, Muslims, Crusaders, French and English all have taken turns occupying this 120-square-mile island. Only beginning in 1964 has the island been ruled by the native Maltese. All world leaders should visit Malta, if only to be reminded how fleeting power can be.

What most amazed me about Malta were the unknown prehistoric people who somehow lugged 50-ton stones to erect the great temples they built in about 2500 B.C.E. These amazing structures predated the pyramid at Cheops by 500 years!

One of the best features of the trip was the guest lecturers traveling with us, including a professor of comparative religion, an expert on the art and architecture of non-western civilizations, and Dr. Charles Liu, who is associated with the American Museum of Natural History's Astrophysics Department. Before we visited a country, we always had extensive lectures about the sights we would encounter. During my unique 36,000 air-mile journey around the world, they helped me come away with two indelible impressions.

The first occurred during an evening I spent stargazing in Australia's outback. These lectures helped me appreciate that the way we see things depends on where we are looking at them. While I was sitting in the middle of the Australian desert, under a pitch-black sky, what I was seeing in the sky over Australia's Southern/Eastern is the exact opposite of what I usually see in the Northern/Western Hemisphere. I saw the universe in a way I had never seen it before and it was magnificent!

My second set of insights emerged from my visits to so many ancient cultures that had built magnificent structures without the benefit of the wheel. I wondered how the early inhabitants of Easter Island were able to carve, let alone move, their giant prehistoric statues (moai). I was also puzzled by the ability of the Mayan priests at sites such as Tikal and Machu Picchu and the priests at Neolithic sites in Malta to make accurate astronomical projections. Even more astounding, these people had no written language. Suddenly, I realized what all these widely scattered civilizations had in common: they vanished without a trace and we don't know why. Doesn't it make you wonder what will happen to our western civilization? Will it continue to flourish or vanish without a whimper?

The beauty of travel is that it further increases your appreciation of this beautiful planet and helps you understand all the incredible cultures that have come before ours.

Other Resources:

American Association of Retired Persons
www.aarp.org/travel
Webplace Travel area and discussion boards.

Earthwatch
www.earthwatch.org
Provides environmentally conscious programs for volunteers of all ages in many different cultures, such as an archaeological dig in Egypt or helping escort sea turtle hatchlings safely to sea.

Elderhostel
www.elderhostel.org
Offers education and adventures for adults 55 and over, including several travel packages for grandparents and grandchildren.

Grandtravel
www.grandtrvl.com
Specializes in guided educational trips in the U.S. and abroad for grandparents and grandchildren with teachers on hand to tie trips into school curricula.

Rascals in Paradise
www.rascalsinparadise.com
Organizes family-friendly trips in the U.S. and around the world.

United States National Park Service
www.nps.gov
The United States National Parks have camping and hiking opportunities and many structured ranger-led programs for various age groups.

Chapter 10

*Living to Be 100:
How to Take Charge and Take Care of Ourselves*

Centenarians—people aged 100 and older—are the fastest-growing group of older Americans. By the year 2050, approximately 834,000 Americans are projected to have celebrated their 100th birthday, according to the 2000 Census.

Public health measures such as widespread availability of clean drinking water, nationwide vaccination efforts and the systematic reduction of maternal and childhood mortality rates have helped us live to riper old ages. So have effective treatments for heart disease, pneumonia, diabetes and many types of cancer.

But what's so great about increased longevity? Why live to be 80, 90 or 100 just to feel old? "We survive because we must, because it is inevitable, and because it is possible to enjoy life and its pleasures, and at the same time, make contributions to our fellow human beings," writes Robert Butler in the new preface to his reissued book, *Why Survive? Being Old in America* (Johns Hopkins University Press, 2003).

Butler, founding director of the National Institute on Aging and president of the International Longevity Center in New York, coined the term "ageism" in 1968. He says major health gains help redefine what it means to be old. When Butler was admitting people to nursing homes in the 1950s, he recalls, "We were admitting people on average at age 65. Today it's 81." People today are more active, and biologically, we don't really begin to be old until we're in our eighties or nineties.

But why do some of us age so well and others suffer and die earlier? Contrary to common beliefs, genes have little to do with longevity. Recent research reveals that only 30 percent of the characteristics of aging are genetically determined. The other 70 percent are linked to our state of mind and lifestyle.[1]

However, after age 80, genetics plays an increasingly important role in determining which people survive to 100. "To get to 100, to go the extra

20 years or so, I'd say you need these special genes, these genetic booster rockets," says Thomas T. Perls, author of *Living to 100: Lessons in Living to Your Maximum Potential at Any Age* (Basic, 1999).

This chapter will focus on what we seniors and soon-to-be seniors can do to maximize our own health.

Our body ages not from overuse, but from disuse. Stanford researcher James F. Fries writes in the *New England Journal of Medicine* that many diseases related to aging result from the cumulative effect of bad habits.

In Dr. Thomas Perl's *New England Centenarian Study*, almost none of the participants had encountered life-threatening cancers. The only chronic disease they suffered was arthritis. On average, the centenarians in the study lived without disability until about age 97 and took only one medication. What a dramatic demonstration of the principle that growing old and becoming ill do not necessarily go together! In fact, after the centenarians in the study died, autopsies showed none of the markers of Alzheimer's disease-plaques and tangles in the brain. This exciting discovery means that aging and Alzheimer's are two separate processes.

The good news is that if you make it past 80 without a major illness, you have a lot more living to do. And when the oldest of the old did finally succumb to ill health, the period of time in which they suffered and died was relatively short. What do we need to do to enjoy a similar fate?

Stay Active

Inactivity is the biggest culprit, accounting for about half of our functional decline between ages 30 and 70. Lack of exercise weakens our muscles, including the most important muscle, the heart. Inactivity also contributes to obesity and joint disorders.

The generation now in its fifties, who created the fitness revolution in the 1970s, is hitting the treadmill with a new purpose. This is due, in large part, to studies that show that regular exercise has a positive effect both on one's health and one's physical appearance.

But the type of exercise boomers are doing differs from the type they did in their younger years. They are wisely passing up knee-pounding and muscle-grinding activities in favor of gentler, low-impact exercises. Older Americans are signing up for Tai Chi with three-pound weights, water aerobics and new forms of yoga such as "power yoga" that mix flexibility with cardiovascular benefits.

Exercising at home has also grown in popularity. Boomers have helped push spending on home gym equipment to $5.9 billion in 2001. The most popular items: treadmills, stationary bicycles and elliptical trainers (the latest cardiovascular machines that allow you to have a nearly impact-free aerobic workout) designed to stimulate activity without strain.

Of course you don't have to shell out big bucks for fancy equipment to work out effectively at home. Many people have purchased low-tech medicine balls, elastic bands and vinyl stability balls that improve strength and flexibility without creating bulging muscles.

Eat Well, But Not Too Much

Indeed, if you are what you eat, what can we conclude about those who are 100-plus? When they were growing up, at the turn of the 20th century, diets were quite fatty and heavily salted. Fresh fruit was rare. On the plus side, processed food did not exist. The most striking factor may be that they ate varied diets, and consumed small portions. Dr. Perl found that 99% of the centenarians he studied were not obese.

Yet obesity is very much a problem for about 61% of the rest of the population. The problem has a lot to do with the traditional food pyramid, which overemphasizes carbohydrates. Portions at fast-food and most other kinds of restaurants have gotten progressively bigger.

I recently interviewed actress Suzanne Somers on my radio show, *A Touch of Grey*. She insisted, "It's not fat that makes you fat, but the excess sugar, which turns into cholesterol." A breast cancer survivor in her late fifties, Somers recalled how she put on 20 pounds in her forties even though she hadn't changed her diet or exercise regimen. "I used to watch my French friends and ask why are they so skinny? They were eating salad dressing and cheese and cream. That's when I started looking at the food combining, and that led me to endocrinologist Dr. Schwartzbein," explained Somers, also of thigh-master fame and author of Suzanne Somers' *Eat, Cheat and Melt the Fat Away* (Crown Pub., 2001). By the time she was diagnosed with breast cancer in 2000, she says she was already eating right. She credits her more healthful diet with her ability to beat the cancer even though after surgery and radiation she opted against chemotherapy in favor of a complementary drug called Iscador, which uses extracts of mistletoe. This drug has been used in Europe and Asia but has not undergone clinical trials in the United States. Her decision stirred up some controversy when she announced her experience on Larry King Live on CNN. Many doctors feared that other patients might decide to follow Somers' example, which might not work for them.

Her cancer controversy aside, you can find helpful information about fitness, beauty and diet on her website, www.suzannesomers.com.

Dr. Edward Schieder, dean of the Andrus Gerontology Center at the University of Southern California, suggests this daily "Formula for Longevity" to help prevent diseases and disorders associated with aging:

Vitamin C	200 milligrams
Vitamin E	200 milligrams
Vitamin B	12 milligrams
Vitamin D	400 International Units
Folic Acid	30 grams
Water	8 glasses

Boomers, who grew up distrusting authority figures including doctors, have embarked on an anti-aging quest for healthy food, herbal remedies and nutritional supplements. According to *American Demographics* magazine, boomers dominate the $28 billion market for food and drinks that incorporate nutritional supplements in their products, such as nutraceuticals like Actimel, a drink made by Danone that has bacterial cultures that help fortify the body's immune system. Then there are cereals that are fortified with antioxidants.

Constantly seeking their own health answers and alternative treatments, boomers have taken to herbs such as ginkgo and elderberries for mental clarity, and glucosamine to keep their joints limber. They also seek their fountain of youth in a bottle of fitness water or juice, packed with minerals, electrolytes and vitamins. Perfect for those on the run!

Cope with Stress

The lives of the centenarians in the study were not necessarily easy. They experienced their share of problems, such as poverty, hardship, oppression and personal loss. Their longevity seemed to result not from having avoided stress, but from having found effective ways of dealing with it. Resilience and an optimistic outlook were their key lifelong personality traits. These people were able to separate themselves from loss and move on. Dr. John Rowe, in his book *Successful Aging* (Dell Publishing Company, 1999), says that centenarians are natural stress shedders who can shrug off life's slings and arrows with relative ease.

Find Supportive Relationships

Four in five of the centenarians are female. Researchers suspect that mutual assistance pacts that women naturally develop provided both comfort and companionship.

Peter Martin of Iowa State University in Ames and his colleagues have found that about 25% to 30% of centenarians no longer have any siblings or children still living, but they often have extended family or close, long-term friends on whom they can rely for support. Martin says that although many studies of centenarians have not examined the role of family support, he believes it plays an important role in the longevity and health of the oldest old.

Don't Ignore Chronic Pain

Aging may increase the risk of experiencing chronic pain—defined as pain that lasts longer than a couple of months. Chronic pain can be constant or recurring, and can vary in intensity. Dr. Paul Ruggieri states in *The Surgery Handbook: A Guide to Understanding Your Operation* (Addicus Books, 1999) that nearly half of post-surgical pain has been under-treated. As well, *Time* magazine reported that 43% of older Americans suffering from joint, back, foot and muscle pain did not feel they had a great deal of control over their pain. Only when their pain became completely unbearable did they even seek a doctor's help. Much of their pain was unnecessary. And, as we'll see, pain can be more than uncomfortable; it can also erode our health.

It is a myth that pain must be a natural part of aging. New pain research shows that chronic pain often becomes a vicious cycle: pain creates stress, which, in turn, magnifies the pain.

While most physicians received little, if any, training in pain management in medical school, the subject is receiving a lot more attention in research and continuing education for physicians. As a result, doctors better understand pain drugs, such as opiates. In the past, doctors often withheld this drug from patients in pain because of addiction fears. Doctors now know that less than 1% of pain patients using narcotic drugs will experience withdrawal problems. Doctors are also using drugs initially intended for other purposes, such as Neurontin, which was developed for epilepsy.

Sixty-something actress Donna Mills told *A Touch of Grey* that she was devastated when she was diagnosed with arthritis several years ago. An avid tennis player, the portrayer of conniving Abby Cunningham of *Knots Landing* recalled that "the problem with pain is pain will take away your sense of humor pretty fast. When I was in pain all the time, I was cranky. It affects your personality. Particularly with something like arthritis, you can't see it, so it's hard for loved ones to understand it."

I, too, have a little arthritis. One thing that helps me is exercise—weight training, aerobic movement and stretching. It's keeping my arthritis at bay. It is also important to keep your mind active with a bunch of projects.

More health professionals are also becoming increasingly aware of the growing number of non-chemical treatments for chronic pain, such as relaxation techniques (yoga and biofeedback), acupuncture, physical therapy, occupational therapy and counseling. Transcutaneous electrical nerve stimulation (TENS) has can help relieve chronic pain from bursitis and osteoarthritis. And surgeons can sometimes block pain-carrying nerves in some patients.

Things you can do:

• **Keep a pain diary,** describing the frequency, intensity and type of pain (throbbing, gnawing or stabbing), what seems to trigger it and whether rest or exercise relieves it. To obtain the proper diagnosis, it's important to give your doctor even the most trivial details about your pain.

- **Find a doctor** who has been certified by the American Board of Pain Medication for an evaluation.

- **Don't be passive.** Don't just quietly accept whatever treatment your doctor prescribes; ask what other options are available, and make sure your doctor informs you about side-effects as well as the benefits of any treatment.

Some further resources on chronic pain:

Living Creatively With Chronic Illness, by Joyce Dace-Lombard and Eugenie G. Wheeler (Pathfinder Publishing of California, 1989)

Managing Pain Before it Manages You, by Margaret Caudill (Guilford Publications, 2001)

A World of Information on Pain
www.pain.com

Arthritis Foundation
www.arthritis.org

The American Chronic Pain Association
www.theacpa.org

Sleep Well

The widely held misconception is that sleeping less is part of getting old. In fact, your sleep needs remain constant throughout your life. If you required seven to nine hours of sleep a night when you were young, you will still require the same amount of sleep when you're older. Sleep scientists are now saying it's not the need for sleep that changes as we age, it's our ability to sleep well and long enough that changes.

In fact, by the time you turn 65, you have a 50% chance of suffering from a chronic sleep problem. Beginning with middle age, your time clock, or circadian rhythms, get pushed forward. The result is the early-to-bed, early-to-rise pattern. You may still get your seven or eight hours of sleep, but at very different hours. One problem is that if your body clock tells you to go to bed at 8:00 pm, you may have to struggle to stay up later for special evening events.

As people get older, other changes in circadian rhythms can result in people sleeping lighter and having staggered periods of wakefulness.[2] The two deepest sleep stages that are the most refreshing and where healing takes place are harder to achieve. This can prevent people from waking up feeling refreshed and make them tired later in the day. If they take a nap, it can further mitigate against establishing a solid sleeping pattern.

But there is good news. Scientists are finding that exposure to light can reset the circadian rhythms of older adults. It turns out, older people spend less time outdoors. And eye diseases such as cataracts may block out the light needed to maintain healthier sleep patterns. As little as two hours of sunlight a day will help you sleep better.

Several medical disorders can also affect senior sleeping. For instance, apnea frequently goes undetected and can be life threatening. With this sleep disorder, one's breathing is temporarily interrupted, sometimes more than 300 times a night, waking the person repeatedly. Another sleep disorder is periodic limb movement, also called restless leg syndrome. It involves feeling unpleasant tingling sensations in the legs, and the urge to shake them frequently, which can impede getting and staying asleep. But both these conditions can be effectively treated, once diagnosed.

Chronic health conditions such as arthritis, heartburn, osteoporosis, heart and pulmonary disease, can also interrupt, delay or shorten the sleep cycle. For instance, medications for treating asthma contain stimulants.

The very drugs for treating insomnia can create new sleep problems. Sedatives help small or temporary sleep problems, but tolerance to the drug may develop, causing the drug to lose effectiveness. When going off the medication, many people experience nightmares, and insomnia may rebound. Worst of all, sleeping medications and tranquilizers have been linked to falls and hip fractures.

But you don't have to be among the 40% of people older than 60 who say they sleep poorly. How well you sleep as you age depends to a large extent on your lifestyle. If you are getting less than the restful 40 winks you require, try some of these strategies:

• **Get more physical exercise.** Dr. Gregg of the Sleep Disorders Clinic of Beth Israel Deaconess Medical Center says you should exercise late in the day before dinner, but at least three hours before bed time.

• **Cut back on caffeine and alcohol**, and avoid both prior to bed time.

• **Don't smoke.** Nicotine is a stimulant!

• **Avoid sleeping pills.** If you do use them, never do so for more than three days in a row.

• **Make your bedroom a good place to sleep.** It should be cool, dark, quiet and well ventilated.

• **Go to bed at a regular time each night** and get up at the same time each morning.

• **Don't read or watch television in bed.** If you use your bedroom just for resting (and, of course, sex!), and if you only go to bed when you are tired, you will sleep better. If you lie awake more than 10 minutes, get up and do something quiet until you're sleepy.

• **If you must get up to go to the bathroom at night, turn on the dimmest light possible.** Light triggers your body to stop producing melatonin, the hormone that helps you sleep.

• **Make getting good sound sleep a priority.** It nurtures both your body and brain.

• **If you have not been able to pinpoint the cause of sleeplessness, con-sider going to a sleep disorder center that can help diagnose the problem. The American Academy of Sleep Medicine's website (www.aasm-net.org/listing.asp) can help you locate an accredited center.

Some good references on sleep:

Sleep Disorders: An Alternative Medicine Guide, by Herbert Ross D.C. and Keri Brenner (National Book Network, 2000)

"In Search of Sleep," *Newsweek*, July 15, 2002.

Limit Alcohol Use

Most people would be surprised to learn the extent of the "invisible epidemic"—the growing number of older Americans with serious drinking problems. In the United States, according to the third edition of *The Encyclopedia of Aging*, an estimated 2.5 million older adults have problems related to alcohol and 21% of hospitalized people over 40 have a diagnosis of alcoholism. When it comes to the 60-plus population, a recent article in the *Elder Law Journal* of the University of Illinois reported that at as many as one in six were overly dependent on alcohol.

Alcohol problems in the elderly are characterized in two ways. The vast majority of senior alcohol abusers fall into the "early-onset" category. This means they have a life-long history of drinking to excess and have already experienced all the emotional, social and physical problems that accompany this disease. About one third of older people who abuse alcohol are part of "late-onset" group. Major life changes and stresses often trigger increased use of alcohol later in life, such as retirement, children leaving home, spouses and friends dying and poor health, which results in physical pain and the lack of mobility. Unlike younger people who begin drinking to be with friends, older people often start, or greatly increase, their drinking because they feel alone and abandoned. Women are more prone than men to late-onset alcoholism. Alcohol becomes the only trusted friend they have.

I was surprised to learn that late-onset alcohol problems also pop up for the first time in retirement communities where drinking at social gatherings is the norm and is greatly encouraged.

Alcohol has a much more damaging effect on an older person's body than a younger person's. This is because aging interferes with the body's ability to metabolize and eliminate alcohol. While a 30-year-old may feel little effect from two drinks, a 70-year-old is much more likely to become intoxicated. Older women generally feel the effects of drinking more than men, because they have a lower amount of body water and are smaller in size. Many older people also suffer a variety of medical problems such as diabetes, heart disease, liver disease, and central nervous system degeneration, conditions that increase the effect alcohol has on the body.

Dr. Jeanne Wei in *Aging Well* (Wiley, 2001) states that up to 15% of Americans over 65 will develop an alcohol problem after the death of a spouse. The dangerous mixture of alcohol with certain medications, both over the counter and prescription, has resulted in a lot of hospital admissions.

With so many older people having problems related to alcohol, why haven't we heard more about it? The main reason is that employers and the police are less likely to come in contact with seniors with this problem, because they are less likely to be working or driving. Another factor is that seniors, who are largely homebound, often drink in isolation. Family members of older adults who know they are drinking too much often don't know what to do about it, or are simply too embarrassed to get help.

Even doctors often misdiagnose alcoholism as depression, anxiety, diabetes or some other problem associated with aging. Also, during brief doctor's visits, patients and their families may place greater emphasis on tangible health problems, such as heart or stomach problems, rather than on potential substance abuse.

Signs of possible alcohol abuse can include changes in sleeping and eating patterns, malnutrition, poor hygiene, tremors, shakiness and frequent falls and bruising—symptoms that, of course, can also be caused by other medical problems.

Alcohol can make some medical problems harder to diagnose. For example, alcohol causes changes in the heart and blood vessels that can dull pain that might warn of a heart attack. Alcohol can also cause forgetfulness and confusion, mimicking Alzheimer's disease. For these very important reasons, family members displaying any of these symptoms need to see a doctor right away.

The only way to get a handle on this insidious disease is to have alcohol screening become part of every older adult's annual physical. Doctors should tell patients the guidelines for drinking for men and women 65-plus: no more than one drink a day. More than three drinks per occasion, two or more times in a month is considered binge drinking.

What about treatment? The good news is that older adults can have as much or more success in reducing or eliminating alcohol from their lives as younger people. The bad news is that very few programs are designed specifically for the older person with alcohol problems. Even when properly diagnosed, seniors often lack a vital support system when they are in treatment. Long-time friends and children have often moved far away.

The cost of alcohol treatment is another problem. Turning to the government for help is not a viable alternative. Medicare will cover the cost of alcohol detoxification, but will not cover a hospital stay for rehabilitation if a less expensive setting is available. Government-reimbursed alcohol treatment, in fact, rarely lasts more than two weeks.

Once older problem drinkers do decide to seek help, they usually stay with their chosen program and do quite well. Getting the proper information and knowing where to turn for treatment is the key to recovery.

If the drinking of someone close to you is creating problems, Al-Anon is a free, confidential source of help. Most cities and towns have Al-Anon groups that meet frequently.

Some excellent resources:

• **The National Council on Alcohol and Drug Information Hotline** can refer you to alcohol treatment services in your area: 800-729-6686.

• **The National Institute on Aging Information Center** has a number of excellent pamphlets on aging and alcohol abuse: 800-222-2225.

• **Alcoholics Anonymous** can help you find a local group and provides lots of helpful information for alcoholics and their family members. It's free and confidential: www.alcoholics-anonymous.org.

Good health habits obviously have a tremendous impact on maximizing the disease-free portion of your life. In addition to the above, today's pioneers of aging recommend the following regimen:

• **Don't smoke.**

• **Keep blood pressure under control.**

• **Keep your mind active** with new and different activities to exercise different parts of your brain.

The real key to living a long life lies in your attitude about aging. The centenarians who participated in the study certainly refused to consider their age a limitation. They remained actively engaged with life.

What is the likelihood that you will live to be 100? You can find out by using the Life Expectancy Calculator at http://www.beeson.org/living-to100/default.htm. The quiz includes questions you might expect about use of tobacco and alcohol, types of foods you eat, stress and exercise, plus some surprising questions about whether or not you floss, exposure to second-hand smoke, radon, sun and polluted air.

Other Resources:

Alive and Well: The Emergence of the Active Nonagenarian, by William F. Powers (Rutledge Books, 1996).

Breaking the Rules of Aging, by Dr. David A. Lipschitz (Lifeline Press, 2002).

Living to 100: Lessons in Living to Your Maximum Potential at Any Age, by Thomas T. Perls, M.D., Margery Hunter Silver Ed. D. and John F. Lauerman (Basic Books, 2000).

Successful Aging, by John W. Rowe, M.D, and Robert L. Kahn, Ph.D. (Delacorte Press, 1999).

Chapter 11

*Nothing to Sneeze At:
Navigating the Health-Care System*

How can we best access our over-burdened, over-regulated, over-priced health-care system to get the best care?

That's not an easy task, especially with the Medicare Reform Act, which Congress passed just before Thanksgiving 2003 by a razor-thin margin. Figuring out how to find the best health care requires the agility and skill of a sailor navigating a turbulent sea. I don't have all the answers, but drawing on my personal experiences, research and interviews with some experts, this chapter offers some guidance and moral support that can help you ride the waves with more confidence.

First, let's get a sense of what we're up against.

Kiplinger's newsletter forecasts that by 2011, health care will claim an amazing 12% of this country's gross national product.

The United States has a medical system largely based on private insurance plans. But by 2030, Medicare will be the primary insurer for one in every four Americans. As a result, we can expect to face tough Medicare and health-care choices as the age wave surges. And while the new Medicare Reform Act will potentially help many older Americans, those health-care choices are tougher to understand than ever.

Medicare Reform Act: Will You Be a Winner or Loser?

There will most certainly be winners and losers. But the 1,100-page legislation is so complex that it will take years for Medicare beneficiaries, as well as health-care experts, to sort it out. I'm not so sure all the senators and congressmen who passed this law have read and understood all its provisions.

Among the winners:

• Some 13.4 million poor elderly and those who pay more than $5,100 a year out of their own pocket for prescription drugs—but not until 2006, when the new drug benefits take effect. In the meantime, as of the spring of 2004, Medicare beneficiaries are able to purchase a card for about $30 that will trim an estimated 10% to 15% off prescriptions.

• Seniors with chronic diseases such as diabetes, asthma, hypertension and congestive heart failure will find coverage to manage those conditions, and for preventive measures and early diagnosis.

• Drug companies, health insurers and employers are slated to receive about $125 billion over the next years in direct assistance and tax breaks.

Losers include:

• Middle-income people—those who earn more than $80,000 a year and have more than $6,000 in assets (excluding the value of their homes and their cars—if used for work or medical visits), will not be eligible for subsidies for their Medicare premiums, which come to $425 a year. In fact, Kaiser projects that the average senior who takes out that estimated premium and pays the deductible will pay out of pocket $1,500.

• 48 million baby boomers, who will be in or near their seventies by 2026, the year recent federal estimates expect Medicare will become insolvent. The new law makes no effort to contain costs—there are no provisions for cheaper drugs from Canada or Europe, or provisions to negotiate, as the Veterans Administration does, with pharmaceutical companies for better prices. How crazy is it that our government won't be able to negotiate a better price on its $400 billion spending on drugs for 40 million seniors?

One study found that 31% of seniors who knew little about the bill opposed it. Opposition jumped to 54% among seniors who were educated about the bill's main provisions. If more people find out the details, there may well be a backlash. Some seniors ripped up their membership cards to the Association of American Retired Persons (AARP) after that organization endorsed the Medicare Bill. Obviously AARP has a conflict of interest because it has such a big insurance program, which is a profit-making entity, and also has a drug benefit program. AARP should not have taken a stand.

I don't think there's any question that Medicare needed reform. The question is, will the kind of reforms just passed be appropriate reform?

Health-Care Rationing

And what does the future hold? Will the medical system explicitly ration health care in the face of overwhelming medical costs, increasing need for treating Americas as they live longer and dwindling resources to meet this need? Will age become a basis for rationing of health care? This is a scary thought, but not necessarily unrealistic, when you consider:

• The fastest-growing segment of our population is 85 years and older.

• Half of this age group will develop the costly and chronic Alzheimer's disease, not to mention other chronic illnesses.

• One-third of all Medicare spending goes to patients in the last years of life.

As a result, health-care in the 21st century will pose excruciatingly tough choices, such as:

• Marvelous and expensive life-extending technologies are available, but who will be allowed to benefit from these modern miracles, such as stem cell and organ transplants?

• Should age, cost of a specific treatment or the probability of survival be factored into who lives and who dies?

• Who should decide these important ethical and moral questions?

Although there may be no way to provide all the health care an aging society needs and wants, one very practical policy should and could be initiated: make chronic disease prevention, treatment and self-care a national priority. As I described above, the recent Medicare reforms make progress in this area, covering preventive measures such as early diagnosis. But by and large, our present medical system revolves around diagnosing and treating acute diseases. This strategy has worked so well that we have produced legions of long-lived adults, many of whom suffer chronic diseases. We need to educate and train more health-care professionals to meet the needs of today's older Americans.

In the meantime, we need to find, or become our own, health care advocates. Rule number one is not to take doctors' words as gospel.

When to Question, When to Comply

If you're 50-plus you need to ask yourself if the drugs you're taking do more harm than good. Last year, the *Journal of the American Medical Association* reported that medications prescribed to nearly 7 million older Americans—about one-fifth of the population age 65 or older—are rarely appropriate for people their age. The dosage prescribed is also often incorrect. The result: a huge number of adverse drug reactions, many of which require hospitalization.

The two main problems:

• In all U.S. medical schools, pediatric care is mandatory, but geriatric care, if taught at all, is glossed over. Only three of the 144 medical schools in this country have full departments in geriatrics, and only 12 require students to take courses in geriatrics, according to the International Longevity Center.

• Few of the most common drugs that older adults take are ever tested on them, according to Dr. Sidney M. Wolfe, the lead author of *Worst Pills, Best Pills* (Pocket, 1999).

The recommended dosage for most medications is based on a 154-

pound man with normal metabolism. No allowance is given for age (or the female gender). However, with age, the human body has less muscle mass, slower metabolism and develops a greater sensitivity to many drugs. Two important organs, the liver and kidney, become less able to process drugs and clear them from the body. The fact that many older adults suffer from more than one disease is a prescription for disaster. The more diseases one has, inevitably, the more prescribed drugs that person is likely to be taking, and the greater the likelihood for adverse reactions and interactions.

Tip: Before your doctor writes you a prescription, ask: Is this the proper dose for my age and weight?

The fact that older adults have an increased sensitivity to drugs is particularly troubling, especially when it comes to the class of drugs that act on the nervous system. Taken at the same dosage as a young person, tranquilizers for example, can accumulate in an older person's body at dangerously high levels and for longer periods of time. Being overly sedated can lead to tragic falls and hip fractures.

Some older adults' deaths during a heat wave could be attributed to drugs that interfere with the body's temperature regulation. It is well known that as you grow older, it becomes harder for your body to withstand temperature extremes.

To protect yourself, follow these four suggestions:

1. Educate yourself about the medicines you're taking. Each year have several medication reviews with your primary care doctor or pharmacist. Be sure to mention any over-the-counter medications you might be taking.

2. To find out more about the adverse ways drugs can interact, read the book, *Worst Pills, Best Pills*, by Dr. Sidney M. Wolfe (Pocket, 1999).

3. Make sure that once you are confident you have been prescribed the proper medication and dose, that you follow your doctor's orders. Indeed, some patients sometimes contribute to their own medication woes by ignoring doctors' orders and take prescribed medications irregularly, if at all. The reasons patients give for stopping—or never starting—taking medications vary. Some simply forget. Others lack money or insurance. Some

can't tolerate the side effects. If the latter is the case, it's very important to let your doctor know immediately, so the dose or medicine itself can be altered.

Many people take their medications haphazardly. I've been there, done that and I can tell you that this behavior can lead to even more health problems. For instance, several years ago I was prescribed antibiotics for an infection. I took the pills for four or five days and felt better, so I stopped taking the pills. Then my symptoms reappeared much worse. So I learned that you need to complete the full course of treatment. Now I'm a patient who questions and then complies. Be one too!

Avoiding Preventable Medical Errors

It may sound cynical, but in some cases, we might be better off being blocked from receiving medical care. After all, preventable medical errors are the eighth leading cause of death in America! Between 44,000 and 98,000 people die each year in U.S. hospitals from mistakes made by medical professionals, according to the National Academy of Science's Institute of Medicine.

And that might be a conservative estimate, according to Dr. Donald Berwick of the Institute of Medicine. He believes that many errors are never written down, much less reported. He also points out that the current medical errors study didn't include other important areas in the health care system where mistakes can be made, such as ambulatory clinics, outpatient surgery centers, doctors' offices, nursing homes, pharmacies and patients' homes.

Medication errors are among the most widespread type of preventable medical mistakes. For instance, a patient might receive the wrong prescription or dosage.

Tip: When your doctor writes a prescription, make sure you can read it and know what it is for!

Name confusion is among the most common causes of drug-related errors. Ever wonder why so many drugs have names that sound alike?

Tip: When you pick up your prescription from your pharmacist, ask him or her to check that this is the medicine your doctor ordered!

If you're taking a new drug, find out what adverse reactions have been reported.

Tip: Buy a copy of the *Physician Desk Reference* (Thomson Healthcare, 2002), which lists side-effects and other important information about medicines.

This literally saved my life when I had an adverse reaction to Lipitor, a cholesterol-lowering drug. When I started feeling a crushing pressure in my chest and had difficulty breathing, I realized these are also symptoms of a heart attack, so I was quite nervous. I looked up the medication in the PDR, which, buried in there, listed those symptoms, and I relaxed. But in the middle of the night it got much worse, so I called 911. I told them what I had read about the Lipitor I was taking, but they insisted that I have a complete work up. All the tests were negative, but I learned that it's important when you're starting any new treatment to find out and discuss with your doctor what the symptoms could possibly be, and what to do if you are experiencing those side effects.

Older patients are at special risk when taking medication, because the aging body, which has less ability to metabolize substances, can react even more strongly than other age groups when experiencing side-effects.

Surgical errors account for a high percentage of medical errors.

Tip: To ensure your surgery has a positive outcome, choose a hospital (if you can) at which many patients have had the same type of procedure.

Other medical errors include making the wrong diagnosis, giving patients the wrong blood type, post-surgical wound infection and misinterpretation of someone else's medical orders.

Tip: Have your personal doctor take charge of your overall care while you are in the hospital, especially if you have many health problems.

We've all heard of wrong-site surgery—it's rare, but should be 100% preventable. The American Academy of Orthopedic Surgeons urges its members to sign their initials directly on the site to be operated on before surgery.

Tip: Make sure you, your doctor and your surgeon all agree and are clear on exactly what will be done.

The Institute of Medicine points to the Veterans Administration health-care system as an example of how to reduce medical errors. The VA has improved its medication safety record by using a new bar-coding system to prevent and track medical errors. Nurses, patients and medication containers all wear identification strips. Before giving a patient a drug, a nurse scans all three ID strips into a computer, which verifies that the drug is given correctly and will not cause negative interactions with other medications. VA hospitals that used this system reduced medication errors by 70% in five years.

The Institute of Medicine also suggests laws that would require hospitals—and later clinics, doctors' offices and nursing homes—to report to state officials any deaths or serious injuries caused by medical errors. Information on less serious errors would be kept confidential to encourage voluntary compliance. Of course doctors and hospitals fear that mandatory reporting would open them up to more malpractice suits. Nonetheless, the Institute of Medicine urged Congress to create a National Center for Patient Safety within the Department of Health and Human Services, to act as a clearinghouse for information on patient safety nationwide, and to fund research to find better ways to prevent errors.

Unfortunately, so far Congress has not acted on these practical suggestions. But consumers can and should take responsibility in several areas:

• Consumer education is key.

• Be vigilant about your health care and any treatments doctors prescribe.

• Keep organized records of any doctor visits and medications you take.

• Above all, be persistent and ask questions, especially when things don't seem right.

Here are further resources on preventing medical errors:

Agency for Healthcare Research and Quality
www.ahcpr.gov

"Twenty Tips to Help Prevent Medical Errors"
800-358-9295

When Your Doctor Doesn't Know Best: Medical Mistakes That Even the Best Doctors Make—And How to Protect Yourself, by Dr. Richard N. Podell, (Simon & Schuster, 1995).*

Doctor Generic Will See You Now: 33 Rules for Surviving Managed Care, by Dr. Oscar London, (Ten Speed Press, 1996).*

*These are out of print, but copies can likely be found in many libraries or at online used bookstores.

Getting an Early Diagnosis

Many common diseases go undiagnosed for a long time. The longer a disease is untreated, the more damage it is likely to do. Here are three examples of some very common, and unpleasant, health problems that may defy easy detection:

• **Irritable Bowel Syndrome.** One in five people suffers from the severe abdominal pain, bloating and constipation, alternating with diarrhea that IBS causes. Although this disease can affect people of all ages, 70% of the sufferers are women. Even Wonder Woman's mother is not immune. Actress Lynda Carter told *A Touch of Grey* recently that her mother had it for 30 years, but suffered for 15 years before being diagnosed.

So far, no blood or stool, x-ray, ultrasound or any other diagnostic test can definitively diagnosis IBS. Doctors can only make a diagnosis based on symptoms (mentioned above) and rule out other conditions.

I was diagnosed 15 years ago after every kind of test to rule out every other kind of disease. It can be aggravated by travel, stress, change in diet or taking new medicine. For instance, after a root canal, I took codeine, which can—and did—cause constipation. IBS sufferers need to be hyper-aware of such side effects before they take new medications!

One big problem is that many patients are embarrassed to discuss these symptoms, even with their doctor. Another barrier to diagnosis is ignorance. While there is plenty of information today, especially on the Internet (see, for instance, the Society for Women's Health Research website www.talkibs.org/index.html), not many doctors are well versed about IBS. "You may be the one informing your doctor," points out Carter, who is in her mid-fifties.

Medicines often just exacerbate this condition. For instance, antispasmodics are used to relieve cramps or spasms of the stomach, intestines and bladder, but may also cause constipation, decreased sweating, dryness of mouth, nose, throat or skin, and, in rare cases, confusion, dizziness, lightheadedness (continuing) or fainting, eye pain, skin rash or hives. While fiber supplements such as Metamucil may help some, a slight change in diet—even water—when an IBS sufferer travels, for instance, can trigger an episode.

- **Chronic Obstructive Pulmonary Disease.** Loni Anderson, who lost both her parents while in their sixties to this killer, has become a spokeswoman to help educate the public.

"A lot of women don't realize they have it," she explained on a recent *A Touch of Grey* show, even though an estimated 15% of the population—30 million Americans—have it. Only a little more than half of them have been diagnosed, and last year COPD killed 119,000 people in this country. In fact, COPD is now the fourth leading cause of death, according to Dr. Dennis Dougherty, professor of medicine and chief of pulmonary and critical care medicine of the University of Kentucky, who appeared on my show with Ms. Anderson. "People don't admit or realize their symptoms early enough—until they've lost 50% of their blood function," he says. For instance, a person suffering shortness of breath is likely to stop activities that cause that symptom and then conclude it was nothing serious.

Most sufferers are smokers, and Dr. Dougherty says it's never too late to benefit from giving up that habit. "If they get tested and quit smoking we can help them breathe a little easier."

You can learn more about COPD at www.thebreathingspace.com.

The lessons: your doctor might not be up to date, you may feel sure your symptoms are "nothing" or you may be too scared or embarrassed to discuss them. But you can alleviate much unnecessary suffering and possibly reclaim years of your life by taking your symptoms seriously, by doing a little digging on the Internet, and insisting that your doctor order every conceivable test to identify whatever is ailing you.

• **Colorectal cancer.** Here's a disease that can cut life short, yet is quite easy to spot, rules Judge Judy Scheindlin of NBC courtroom television fame. Unfortunately, her mother did not catch it in time.

Judge Judy told *A Touch of Grey* recently that although her father, a dentist, was in the medical profession, her family avoided going to doctors unless they experienced very blatant symptoms. "It's like the cobbler's kids have no shoes," she says.

As she learned after her mother died in her fifties, almost two-thirds of those who die from colorectal cancer could have been successfully cured if they had been properly diagnosed early enough.

Many people may avoid getting regular screenings because they wrongly believe that the diagnostic procedure—a colonoscopy—is painful. Judge Judy dispels that myth. Yes, you have to fast for 24 hours and then drink some unpleasant drink, but then you're given a sedative and sleep through the ordeal.

In her case, she says, "I was positive it would be all clear, but when I woke up they had removed several polyps—that was my wakeup call." Now, instead of repeating the test the usual "every 10 years" (as the American Cancer Society guidelines recommend for people 50 and older), she needs to come back in three years. "There's no better gift you can give yourself than taking this test because you can avoid dying from an illness that's a horrible way to go," she warns in her sternest Judge Judy[1] voice.

Tip: Now there is even a less invasive type of exam, called a "virtual colonoscopy," which utilizes "computerized tomography" to spot evidence of colon cancer, as well as coronary artery and lung disease. The test does not require anesthesia. You can learn more about it at the National Cancer Institute (www.cancer.gov/clinicaltrials/results/virtual-colonoscopy 1203).

The Long and the Short of Long-Term Health Care

The largest unfunded liability facing baby boomers and their elderly parents is the cost of long-term care. Most people believe that Medicare will pay for this service. It does not. Medicare only pays for short-term skilled care, usually 100 days. In addition, Medicare will only cover long-term care if you go directly from a hospital to a nursing home.

Another way to pay for long-term care is to qualify for Medicaid—a welfare program financed by the state and federal government. Eligibility rules differ from state to state. In general, if you want to qualify for Medicaid, you must first liquidate a large percentage of your assets to pay for your own healthcare.

Trudy Liberman of *Consumer Reports* states that half of all women and a third of all men who are now 65 will spend time (many of their last years) in a nursing home. The average annual cost is $50,000 and more. In Connecticut, for example, costs can exceed $80,000 a year.

The insurance industry says private long-term care policies are best suited to those whose non-excludable assets, such as their homes, are valued in excess of $200,000, and whose income is $35,000 or more annually.

Premiums vary greatly from company to company. They are based on your age, the benefits you select, and the number of years you want a company to pay for the benefits. Premiums can range from a few hundred dollars a year for a bare-bones policy bought by people in their thirties to tens of thousands of dollars a year for an all-inclusive, inflation-adjusted policy for those in their sixties.

When should you buy a long-term policy? I bought one at 62. I agree with the advice *Consumer Reports* gives. Buy a policy between 55 and 60 if you have a medical condition, such as diabetes, that could become worse over time. By age 60, you should seriously consider this kind of coverage. The later you buy, the more expensive the policy, and the more difficult it may be to find one. Some companies will accept health conditions that others won't. You need to shop around.

Long-term care insurance is one of the most complex and costly insurance products on the market. It's an insurance jungle out there, and you need to know the right questions to ask. A few of them are:

Can the premium go up?

Does the policy exclude existing conditions?

When do benefits begin?

Is there an inflation rider?

Is the policy automatically renewable?

To learn more, you can get free health insurance counseling at your local area agency on aging, or call the ElderCare Locator toll free number: 800-677-1116.

Afterthoughts

Questions for the Future

What are our national priorities going to be in the 21st century? Many of the issues that older Americans are concerned about today will remain their focus in the coming decade, including Social Security, Medicare, health-care costs and other pocketbook issues. But as the number of seasoned citizens continues to grow dramatically, they will become more vocal.

I believe the window for shaping Social Security and Medicare will extend through 2010. After that, it will be very difficult to change these entitlements. This is because the oldest of the baby boomers, those born in 1946, will become eligible for early retirement under Social Security in 2008 and they will be able to draw Medicare benefits starting in 2011. Millions more politically savvy boomers will be following in their footsteps and they certainly will want to protect their benefits.

Quality-of-life issues for America's graying population will also be brought to the forefront of our nation's consciousness. As more insidious forms of health care rationing become a reality, more Americans may find themselves unable to afford expensive new technologies that could extend their lives. By deciding what treatments they will pay for, might traditional Medicare and Medicare HMOs become the final arbitrators of who will live and who will die?

Another question that will loom in the future is how many baby boomers will be able to retire and forego their weekly paycheck? John Goodman, president of the National Center for Policy Analysis, recently testified before the Senate Aging committee that "most people ages 55 to 64, the decade before they qualify for Medicare, have no retirement savings accounts. Even those who have set money aside don't have much. Their median balance is $25,000."

Will there be jobs in the next decade for those older workers who will need them? Will increased globalization and outsourcing of jobs continue to pose long-term challenges for the job market?

The biggest unknown that will affect the well being of all Americans, young and old, will be the state of our nation's deficit. One must wonder how much it will grow in future years. Of course military and national security funding will remain top priorities, as long as worldwide acts of terrorism continue. What we don't presently know is whether fiscal constraints will cause important domestic programs to be down sized.

Our children are our future. Will we see cuts that will affect their education, as well the environment in which they live?

Of course, when it comes to seasoned citizens, I wonder how much future financial support the programs of the federally funded Older Americans Act will receive. Some of the vital services funded by this Act include: meals-on-wheels, respite care, older worker programs and ombudsman services. Currently, there are waiting lists for many of the services the Older Americans Act provides.

Presently, 10.5% of seniors have annual incomes below the poverty level, while another 6.5% have incomes just above poverty. In the years ahead, will we see these numbers rise?

Which domestic programs will be funded and how much money will they receive? Will the young and old flourish together in a truly multi-generational society? I can't look into a crystal ball and give answers to the critical questions I've raised. One thing I can say, though, is that I will continue to write about and discuss them!

Resources

ADVOCACY/EDUCATION

A Touch of Grey - Online Resource for Grownups
Additional resources can be found at:
www.atouchofgrey.com

AARP
Nonprofit membership organization for persons 50 and older.
601 E. Street, NW
Washington, DC 20049
888-OUR-AARP
www.aarp.org

Administration on Aging
Promoting consumer awareness, preventing elder victimization and working to implement community partnerships to prevent Medicare and Medicaid fraud, error and abuse.
Washington, DC 20201
202-619-0724
www.aoa.gov

Alliance for Aging Research
Citizen advocacy organization for improving the health and independence of Americans as they age. Offers free publications including "Investing in Older Women's Health," "Meeting the Medical Needs of the Senior Boom," "Delaying the Diseases of Aging" and other aging-related subjects such as menopause, how to age with ease and health-care options under Medicare.
2021 K Street, NW, Suite 305
Washington, DC 20006
202-293-2856
www.agingresearch.org

American Museum of Natural History
A brief overview on aging, the human life cycle and longevity from an anthropological point of view.
Central Park West at 79th Street
New York, NY 10024
212-769-5100
www.amnh.org

American Society on Aging
Nonprofit organization committed to enhancing the knowledge and skills of those working with older adults and their families.
833 Market Street, Suite 511
San Francisco, CA 94103
415-974-9600 or 800-537-9728
www.asaging.org

Better Business Bureau Alerts
Warns against scams targeting seniors. Shopping tips. Tips for wise giving.
4200 Wilson Boulevard, Suite 800
Arlington, VA 22203
www.bbb.org

Global Action on Aging
International grassroots citizen group that works on issues of concern to older people.
PO Box 20022
New York, NY 10025
212-557-3163
www.globalaging.org

HelpAge International
Global network of not-for-profit organizations with a mission to work with and for disadvantaged older people worldwide to achieve a lasting improvement in the quality of their lives.
www.helpage.org

National Association of State Units on Aging
Public-interest organization providing information, assistance and advocacy on behalf of older people.
1201 15th Street NW, Suite 350
Washington, DC 20005
202-898-2578
www.nasua.org

National Committee to Preserve Social Security and Medicare
Advocate for the landmark federal programs of Social Security and Medicare and for all Americans who seek a healthy, productive and secure retirement.
10 G Street, N.E. Suite 600
Washington, DC 20002
202-216-0420
www.ncpssm.org

National Indian Council on Aging
To bring about improved comprehensive services for American Indian and Alaska native elders.
10501 Montgomery Boulevard NE, Suite 210
Albuquerque, NM 87111
505-292-2001
www.nicoa.org

Seniors Coalition
Non-profit, 501c(4), non-partisan, education and issue advocacy organization that represents the interests and concerns of America's senior citizens at both the state and federal levels.
9001 Braddock Road, Suite 200
Springfield, VA 22151
800-325-9891
www.senior.org

Older Women's League (OWL)
Organization to focus solely on issues unique to women as they age.
1750 New York Avenue, NW, Suite 350
Washington, DC 20006
800-825-3695 or 202-783-6686
www.owl-national.org

United Seniors Association
Nonprofit, nonpartisan organization founded in 1991.
3900 Jermantown Road #450
Fairfax, VA 22030
1-800-887-2872 or 703-359-6500
www.usanext.org

U.S. Senate Special Committee on Aging
Serves as a focal point in the Senate for discussion and debate on matters relating to older Americans.
G31 Dirksen Senate Office Building
Washington, DC 20510
202-224-5364
www.senate.gov/~aging

CARE-GIVING

Hospice Foundation of America
Not-for-profit organization that provides leadership in the development and application of hospice and its philosophy of care.
2001 S Street, NW #300
Washington DC 20009
800-854-3402
www.hospicefoundation.org

National Association for Home Care & Hospice
Association publications include *How to Choose a Home Care Provider* and other free consumer guides on home care and hospice care.
228 7th Street, SE
Washington, DC 20003
202-547-7424
www.nahc.org

National Association of Professional Geriatric Care Managers
Non-profit, professional organization of practitioners whose goal is the advancement of dignified care for the elderly and their families.
1604 N. Country Club Road
Tucson, AZ 85716
520-881-8008
www.caremanager.org

National Center on Elder Abuse
National resource for elder rights, law enforcement and legal professionals, public policy leaders, researchers, and the public. The Center's mission is to promote understanding, knowledge sharing and action on elder abuse, neglect and exploitation.
1201 15th Street, NW, Suite 350
Washington, DC 20005
202-898-2586
www.elderabusecenter.org

National Family Caregivers Association
Grass roots organization created to educate, support, empower and speak up for the millions of Americans who care for chronically ill, aged or disabled loved ones.
10400 Connecticut Avenue, #500
Kensington, MD 20895
800-896-3650
www.nfcacares.org

ENTERTAINMENT/TRAVEL

Dancing USA
For those who enjoy or want to learn Ballroom, Latin and Swing dancing.
200 N York Road
Elmhurst, IL 60126
800-290-1307
www.dancingusa.com

Elderhostel
Non-profit educational and travel organization for older adults.
11 Avenue de Lafayette
Boston, MA 02111
877-426-8056
www.elderhostel.org

Ms. Senior Sweetheart Pageant
This pageant was started in 1978 as a Lions' Club fund raiser and is now national. To be a contestant, you must be a female who is age 59 or older.
45 10th Street,
Fall River, MA 02720
508-675-0249
www.msseniorsweetheart.com

Pet Love Shack
Resources for adopting a pet, animal-assisted therapy and pet health.
317 Shewville Road
Ledyard, CT 06339
www.petloveshack.com

National Piano Foundation
The fastest-growing group of aspiring pianists in the U.S. today is not children, but adults aged 25 to 75-plus.
13140 Coit Road, Suite 320, LB 120
Dallas, TX 75240
972-233-9107
www.pianonet.com

National Senior Games Association (NSGA)
NSGA is a community-based member of the United States Olympic Committee and serves as one of the USOC's official arms to the senior population. The NSGA is in charge of conducting the National Senior Games/Senior Olympics. To compete in these games, you must be at least 50 years of age and qualify at a NSGA sanctioned state game.
3032 Old Forge Drive
Baton Rouge, LA 70808
225-925-5678
www.ucp.org

INDEPENDENT/ASSISTED LIVING

ABLEDATA
Sponsored by the National Institute on Disability and Rehabilitation Research, U.S. Department of Education to provide information, assistive technology and rehabilitation equipment.
8630 Fenton Street, Suite 930
Silver Spring, MD 20910
800-227-0216
TTY: 301-608-8912
www.abledata.com

American Association of Homes and Services for the Aging
Nonprofit organization providing older people with services and information on housing, health care and community involvement.
2519 Connecticut Avenue, NW
Washington, DC 20008
202-783-2242
www.aahsa.org

Assisted Living Federation of America (ALFA)
Association exclusively dedicated to the assisted living industry and the population it serves.
11200 Waples Mill Road, Suite 150
Fairfax, VA 22030
703-691-8100
www.alfa.org

Meals on Wheels Association of America
Represents those who provide congregate and home-delivered meal services to people in need.
1414 Prince Street, Suite 302
Alexandria, Virginia 22314
703-548-5558
www.mowaa.org

National Council on the Aging
Founded in 1950, it is a national network of organizations and individuals dedicated to improving the health and independence of the older person.
300 D Street, SW, Suite 801
Washington, D.C. 20024
202-479-1200
www.ncoa.org

National Center for Home Equity Conversion (NCHEC)
Independent, not-for-profit organization dedicated to reverse mortgage analysis and consumer information on reverse mortgages.
360 N Robert #403
Saint Paul MN 55101
651-222-6775
www.reverse.org

National Resource Center on Supportive Housing & Home Modifications
USC Andrus Gerontology Center
3715 McClintock Avenue
Los Angeles, CA 90089
213-740-1364
www.homemods.org

LEGAL

iLawAmerica
A bit unsure about the necessity and practicality of a will?
www.ilawamerica.com

National Academy of Elder Law Attorneys
Non-profit association that assists lawyers, bar organizations and others who work with older clients and their families.
1604 North Country Club Road
Tucson, AZ 85716
520-881-4005
www.naela.org

MEDICAL

Alzheimer's Disease Education and Referral (ADEAR) Center
PO Box 8250
Silver Spring, MD 20907
800-438-4380 (English, Spanish) or 301-495-3311
www.alzheimers.org

Alzheimer's Association
National network dedicated to advancing Alzheimer's research and helping those affected by the disease.
225 North Michigan Avenue, Suite 1700
Chicago, IL 60601
312-335-8700 or 800-272-3900
www.alz.org

Alzheimer's Foundation
John Douglas French
11620 Wilshire Blvd., Suite 270
Los Angeles, CA 90025
800-477-2243 or 310-445-4650
www.jdfaf.org

American Cancer Society
Nationwide, community-based voluntary health organization.
P.O. Box 102454
Atlanta, GA 30368
www.cancer.org

American Heart Association
National Center
7272 Greenville Avenue
Dallas, TX 75231
800-242-8721
www.americanheart.org

Arthritis Foundation (AF)
Nonprofit, volunteer organization focusing on research and information to cure, prevent or better treat arthritis and related diseases.
1330 West Peachtree Street
Atlanta , GA 30309
800-283-7800 or 404-965-7537
www.arthritis.org

Centers for Medicare & Medicaid Services (CMS)
Federal agency within the U.S. Department of Health and Human Services
7500 Security Boulevard
Baltimore MD 21244
877-267-2323
www.cms.hhs.gov

EyeCare America
Public service foundation of the American Academy of Ophthalmology. People with insurance will be billed. Uninsured patients *might* get free care from 7,500 volunteer ophthalmologists across the U.S.
800-391-3937 (EYES)
www.eyecareamerica.org.

Families USA
National nonprofit, non-partisan organization dedicated to the achievement of high-quality, affordable health care for all Americans.
1334 G Street, NW
Washington, DC 20005
202-628-3030
www.familiesusa.org

Lighthouse International
Resources worldwide on vision impairment and vision rehabilitation.
111 East 59th Street
New York, NY 10022
800-829-0500
www.lighthouse.org

Medicare
The Official U.S. Government site for people with Medicare.
www.medicare.gov

National Center for Complementary and Alternative Medicine Clearinghouse (NCCAM)
Provides information on alternative medical therapies not commonly used or previously accepted in conventional Western medicine.
National Institutes of Health (NIH)
PO Box 8218
Silver Spring , MD 20907
888-644-6226 or 301-231-7357
www.nccam.nih.gov

National Coalition for Women with Heart Disease
818 18th Street, NW, Suite 730
Washington, DC 20006
202-728-7199
www.womenheart.org

National Institutes of Health (NIH)
9000 Rockville Pike
Bethesda, MD 20892
http://health.nih.gov

National Osteoporosis Foundation
1232 22nd Street NW
Washington, DC 20037-1292
202-223-2226
www.nof.org

Self Help for Hard of Hearing People
7910 Woodmont Avenue, Suite 1200
Bethesda, MD 20814
301-657-2248
TTY: 301-657-2249
www.shhh.org

Telehealth
5600 Fishers Lane, Room 7C-22
Rockville, MD 20857
301-443-0447
www.telehealth.hrsa.gov

RESEARCH

Duke University Center for the Study of Aging and Human Development
www.geri.duke.edu

International Longevity Center
Not-for-profit, nonpartisan research, policy and education organization whose mission is to help societies address the issues of population aging and longevity in positive and constructive ways and to highlight older people's productivity and contributions to their families and to society as a whole. The ILC-USA is an independent affiliate of Mount Sinai School of Medicine.
60 E. 86th Street
New York, NY 10028
212-288-1468
www.ilcusa.org

National Center on Women & Aging
Focuses on older women's issues and provides policy analysis, research, and assistance to the network of Administration on Aging-funded State and Area Agencies on Aging.
The Heller School for Social Policy and Management
MS 035 Brandeis University
Waltham, MA 02454-9110
1-800-929-1995 or 781-736-3866
http://heller.brandeis.edu/national/index.html

SPRY Foundation
Conducts research and education to help all Americans age successfully.
10 G Street, NE #600
Washington, DC 20002
202-216-0401
www.spry.org

RETIREMENT

Alliance for Retired Americans
A way for retired union members and others to make their voices heard.
888 16th Street, NW, Suite 520
Washington, DC 20006
888-373-6497
www.retiredamericans.org

National Association of Retired Federal Employees (NARFE)
To protect and improve the retirement benefits of federal retirees, employees and their families.
National Headquarters:
606 N. Washington Street
Alexandria, VA 22314
703-838-7760
www.narfe.org

SERVICES

American Geriatrics Society
The Empire State Building
350 Fifth Avenue, Suite 801
New York, NY 10118
212-308-1414
www.americangeriatrics.org

Area Agencies on Aging
Umbrella organization for the 655 area agencies on aging (AAAs) and more than 230 Title VI Native American aging programs in the U.S.
1730 Rhode Island Avenue, NW Suite 1200
Washington, DC 20036
202-872-0888
www.n4a.org

BenefitsCheckUp
The National Council of Aging created this website to help older adults quickly identify Federal and state programs that may improve the quality of their lives.
www.benefitscheckup.org

Department of Veterans Affairs (VA)
1-800-827-1000 to ask a Veteran Services Representative about issues or claims.
www.va.gov

Eldercare Locator
A national toll-free directory assistance public service of the U.S. Administration on Aging that helps people locate aging services in every community throughout the United States.
800-677-1116 Monday through Friday 9:00am to 8:00 pm ET
TDD/TTY: 202-855-1234
(To reach a live operator, dial 202-855-1000. This is not a toll free call.)
www.eldercare.gov

Family Care Giver Alliance
690 Market Street, Suite 600
San Francisco, CA 94104
www.caregiver.org

Gerontological Society of America (GSA)
1030 15th Street, NW, Suite 250
Washington, DC 20005-1503
202-842-1275
www.geron.org

National Adult Day Services Association, Inc.
722 Grant Street, Suite L
Herndon, VA 20170
800-558-5301 or 703-435-8630
www.nadsa.org

National Senior Service Corps
Helps people age 55 and older find service opportunities related to their interests and close to home.
1201 New York Avenue, NW
Washington, DC 20525
202-606-5000
TTY: 202-565-2799
www.seniorcorps.org

Senior Action in a Gay Environment (SAGE)
Social service and advocacy organization dedicated to LGBT (lesbian, gay, bisexual and transgender) seniors.
305 Seventh Avenue, 16th Floor
New York, NY 10001
212-741-2247
www.sageusa.org

Veterans of Foreign Wars of the United States
Enhancing the lives of millions through community service programs and special projects.
National Headquarters
406 West 34th Street
Kansas City, MO 64111
816-756-3390
www.vfw.org

NOTES

Chapter 1

1. Ken Dychtwald, *Age Wave: The Challenges and Opportunities of an Aging America* (J. P. Tarcher; 2000), page 268.
2. *Forbes* magazine's "Top-Paid CEOs" issue, April 15, 2002.

Chapter 3

1. Source: Bureau of Labor Statistics.
2. Dail, P. W. (1988). Prime-time television portrayals of older adults in the context of family life. *The Gerontologist*, 28, 700 - 706.
3. Butler, R., Lewis, M., and Sunderland, T. (1991). *Aging and Mental Health: Positive Psychosocial and Biomedical Approaches*. New York, NY: MacMillan Publishing Company.
4. "Staying Ahead of the Curve: The AARP Work and Career Study," September 2002, http://research.aarp.org/econ/multiwork.html.
5. http://www.aoa.dhhs.gov/factsheets/ageism.html.
6. "7 Fundamental Rules for Crafting a Rock-Solid Resume," by Lance Helgeson, *AARP Bulletin*, September 2002 (http://www.aarp.org/bulletin/departments/2002/life/0905_sidebar_3.html).
7. "8 Interview Questions for Older Workers to Anticipate," *AARP Bulletin*, September 2002. (http://www.aarp.org/bulletin/departments/2002/life/0905_sidebar_4.html).

Chapter 4

1. Joseph F. Coughlin, "Technology Needs of Aging Boomers," *Issues in Science and Technology* Fall 1999, http://www.nap.edu/issues/16.1/coughlin.htm.
2. www.usability.gov.
3. www.aarp.org/olderwiserwired.
4. "Falling Through the Net: Defining the Digital Divide," U.S. Commerce Department, 1997.
5. Section 508 of the Rehabilitation Act Amendments of 1998 requires that when Federal agencies develop, procure, maintain, or use electronic and information technology, they ensure that the electronic and information technology allows disabled Federal employees to access and use information comparable to the access and use non-disabled Federal employees have, unless an undue burden would be imposed on the agency.

Chapter 5

1. http://www.ncoa.org/content.cfm?sectionID=105&detail=43.
2. Lacey Allen, Diane, "A long Life of Love," *The Ledger*, (Lakeland, FL), December 1, 2002. http://www.siecus.org/media/articles/arti0032.html.
3. "Household and Family Characteristics," *Current Population Reports*, March 1998.
4. "The Older Population in the United State," *Current Population Reports*, March 1999.

Chapter 6

1. "Elderly Drivers Die at a Record Pace," *USA Today*.
2. http://www.heller.brandeis.edu/national/shelf.html.
3 "Yoga Trumps Bingo as Centers for Aged Try New Approach," by N. R. Kleinfeld, December 29, 2002.
4 The Baker Medical Research Institute in Melbourne, Australia.

Chapter 7

1. "A New Look at the Old: Grandparents & Aging," University of Cincinnati *E-Briefing*, August 2000.
2. AARP 2002 national survey of 823 grandparents age 50 and older.

Chapter 8

1. Gendell, Murray, "Retirement Age Declines Again in the 1990s," *Monthly Labor Review*, October 2001.
2. *Newsweek* magazine, Dec 16, 2002, page 60.
3. "Planning: The Next Stage," by Jane Bryant Quinn, *Newsweek* magazine, April 3, 2000.
4. ibid.

Chapter 10

1. *Public Citizen Health Letter*, Sidney Wolfe, 1998, www.jrussellshealth.com/convconcerns.html
2. "Special Report: Aging Well," *Wall Street Journal*, Nov. 11, 2002.

Chapter 11

1. Check out her three books: *Don't Pee on My Leg and Tell Me It's Raining* (Perennial, 1997); *Judge Judy Sheindlin's Win or Lose by How You Choose!* (Harper Collins, 2000) and *Judge Judy Sheindlin's You Can't Judge a Book by Its Cover: Cool Rules for School* (Harper Trophy, 2002).